CW00506522

100+ Vegetarian Keto Recipes

2 books in 1:

Delicious Combinations For Keto
Diet With Quick & Healthy Recipes

Anna Prentice

Keto Vegetarian Cookbook

TABLE OF CONTENTS

The 30-Minute Vegetarian Keto Cookbook

TABLE OF CONTENTS

Keto Vegetarian

Cookbook

Amazingly Delicious Vegetarian
Recipes to Living the Keto Lifestyle

Anna Prentice

INTRODUCTION

Do you enjoy cooking and are a fan of the keto diet? If so, the introduction of Vegetarian Keto Cookbook can be an invaluable resource to you. It is an easy-to-follow guide with delicious recipes that are great for anyone who enjoys cooking or wants to learn for the first time. Beginners and experienced chefs alike will find it helpful and full of information that can help them grow their skills in the kitchen.

The Vegetarian Keto Diet is one of the most popular diets right now because of its numerous advantages, including weight loss, blood pressure reduction, diabetes cure, and treatment of other diseases such as cancer. Unlike other diets, this one is full of fat and protein. It has no significant amount of sugar, carbs, or dairy which means that it is easy to be followed for a long time.

Thanks to vegan keto diet, many people are eating better including losing weight. They feel healthier and find it easier to live longer and even get off their medications after getting help from keto diet. The key thing about this diet is that it really results with improved health and a better quality of life. Isn't that wonderful?

To begin, you need to know that there are three kinds of carbohydrates: starch (sugars), sugar, and fiber. Carbs and proteins consist of amino acids which are composed of two types called essential and nonessential amino acids. Some grains also contain a small amount of carbs but the nature is different from other carbs since they do not directly impact blood sugar.

Carbs have a direct impact on blood sugar by raising insulin levels in the body. This can lead to weight gain, type 2 diabetes, and high cholesterol. If you want to lose weight, you need to find ways to reduce your insulin level which means cutting back on carbs or increasing your fat consumption.

Keto is the short form of ketogenic which means that your body will produce ketones in the liver. In case you are wondering, ketones are a source of energy and they're produced by your liver when you deplete your body's carb supply. As much as possible, you should avoid eating carbs in order to force your body to use fat for energy.

When compared to carbohydrates and protein, fat has the least influence on blood sugar, which is why it's crucial to replace carbohydrates with fat. This is known as ketogenesis, and it results in weight reduction and body fat being used as fuel rather than stored as surplus energy.

The ketogenic diet is also a great way to help prevent obesity and type 2 diabetes because it burns fat instead of muscle when someone exercises. This makes them feel fuller faster so they eat less when they're not working out which helps them lose weight more effectively than traditional diets.

The keto diet is also a great way to lose weight because it forces your body to burn fat when you reduce your carbohydrate intake. This type of diet results in lower carb intake, reduced insulin levels, and a lower risk for heart disease. In fact, several studies have indicated that the keto diet can help people lose weight even if they aren't aiming to reduce weight.

RECIPES FOR BREAKFAST

1. Cinnamon Faux Cereal

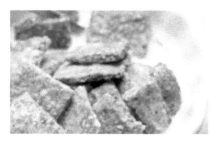

Preparation time: 5 minutes

Cooking time: 25 minutes

Serving: 6 (1/2 cup servings)

Ingredients

- 1 tablespoon of coconut oil
- 1/2 cup of apple cider
- 2 tablespoons of ground cinnamon
- 1/2 cup of hulled hemp seeds
- 1/2 cup of milled flax seed

Directions

1. Preheat the oven to 300 degrees F.
2. Mix all dry ingredients in a food processor, blender or magic bullet. Add the coconut oil and apple cider and process until the ingredients are mostly smooth and fully combined.
3. Spread the batter on a cookie sheet lined with parchment until nice and thin – about 1/16th inch thick
4. Bake in the preheated oven for 15 minutes then lower the heat to 250 degrees and bake for 10 more minutes
5. Remove from oven and cut into squares using a knife or a pizza cutter to about the size of the keys in a computer keyboard

6. Switch off the oven and place the cereal back in the oven until it is completely dried out and crisp.
7. Serve with coconut milk or unsweetened almond milk.

Nutritional info: Calories 129, Protein 9g, Carbs 1.25g and Fat 9g

2. Keto Porridge

Preparation time: 5 minutes

Cooking time: 20 minutes

Serving: 1

Ingredients

- 1 ½ cups of unsweetened almond milk
- 2 tablespoons of vegan vanilla protein powder
- 3 tablespoons of golden flaxseed meal
- 2 tablespoons of coconut flour
- Powdered erythritol to taste

Directions

1. Mix the protein powder, golden flaxseed meal and coconut flour in a bowl
2. Place the above mixture in a saucepan and add the almond milk then cook over medium heat; will appear very loose at first.
3. Stir in your preferred amount of sweetener once it thickens
4. Serve with your favorite toppings

Nutritional info: Calories 249, Protein17.82g, Carbs 5.78g and Fats 13.07g

3. Keto Bread Recipe

Preparation time: 10 minutes

Cooking time: 30 minutes

Serving: 20 slices

Ingredients

- 3 teaspoons of baking powder
- 4 tablespoons of melted butter
- 1 ½ cup of almond flour
- 1 pinch of pink salt
- 6 large eggs, separated
- ½ cup almond flour
- Optional: ¼ teaspoon of cream of tartar
- Optional: 6 drops liquid stevia

Directions

1. Preheat your oven to 375 degrees F.
2. Separate the egg yolks from the egg whites. Add cream of tartar to the egg whites and beat until you achieve soft peaks.
3. Add the melted butter, egg yolks, baking powder, almond flour, salt and 1/3 of the beaten egg whites to the food processor and mix until combined (adding the liquid stevia to the batter helps in reducing the mild egg taste). The resulting mixture will be thick lumpy dough until you add the remaining egg whites
4. Add the rest of the egg whites and process gently until fully incorporated. Ensure you do not over mix the ingredients, as the resulting mixture is what gives the bread its volume
5. Oil an 8x4- inch loaf pan and pour in the mixture. Place in oven and bake for 30 minutes. To ensure the bread is cooked through, check by inserting a toothpick

Nutritional info: Calories 90, Protein 3g, Carbs 2g and Fats 7g

4. Cinnamon Keto Granola

Preparation time: 5 minutes

Cooking time: 20 minutes

Serving: 4

Ingredients

- 4 tablespoons of sugar free maple syrup
- 1.5 oz. nuts (this recipe used almonds, walnuts and pecans)
- 1 tablespoon of chia seeds
- 5 tablespoons of unsweetened coconut flakes
- 5 tablespoons of ground flax meal
- Optional: 1 ½ teaspoons of ground cinnamon

Directions

1. Combine all ingredients apart from the cinnamon.
2. Spread the mixture out onto a baking sheet to form a single layer.
3. Sprinkle the cinnamon on top of the mixture.
4. Bake for 20-22 minutes in the oven at 350 degrees
5. Let it rest, as the granola will harden when it cools. Enjoy

Nutritional info: Calories 175, Protein6g, Carbs 11g and Fats 17g

5. Chia Pudding

Preparation time: 0 minutes

Cooking time: 20-30 minutes

Serving: 1

Ingredients

- 1 tablespoon alcohol free orange extract
- 2-3 tablespoons chia seeds
- 1 cup unsweetened coconut milk
- To make the recipe even tastier there are a couple of additional ingredients that you may consider adding e.g. Blackberries, strawberries, blueberries, cocoa nibs, protein powder, MCT oil, any keto-approved sweetener you like, nuts and nut butters.

Directions

1. Place all ingredients plus any of your desired additional ingredients mentioned above in a bowl or 16 oz. Mason jar. If you are using the jar, put the lid on tight, shake and leave to rest for 20-30 minutes or leave in fridge overnight. If using the bowl, mix all ingredients and the additional ones and let it sit for the above-mentioned time.
2. Your pudding can be anywhere from firm to slightly runny depending on your preference.

Nutritional info: Calories 165, Protein 6g, Carbs 1g and Fat 10.5g

6. Green Coffee Shake

Preparation time: 5 minutes

Cooking time: 0

Serving: 4

Ingredients

- 2 tablespoons of unsweetened almond butter
- 1 1/2 cup of chilled brewed coffee (regular or decaf)
- 1 13.5 fl. oz. (400 ml) can of full-fat coconut milk
- 8 ice cubes, for serving

Directions

1. Add all ingredients apart from the ice cubes to your blender and blend until smooth for around 10 seconds.
2. Divide the shake among four 300 ml (10 fl. Oz.) glasses and drop 2 ice cubes in each glass
3. Enjoy!

Nutritional info: Calories 262, Protein 4.1g, Carbs 4.4g and Fat 24.9g

7. Cauliflower Hash Brown Bowl

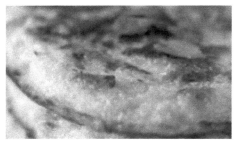

Preparation time: 10 minutes

Cooking time: 10 minutes

Servings: 4

Ingredients:

- 1 cup white mushrooms, chopped
- 1 white onion, diced
- 1 tablespoon coconut oil
- 1 teaspoon pink salt
- 1 teaspoon turmeric
- 1-pound cauliflower, shredded
- 1 teaspoon ground black pepper
- 1 teaspoon garlic powder
- ¼ cup almond milk

Directions:

1. Place the coconut oil in the saucepan.
2. Add chopped mushrooms and diced onion.
3. Sprinkle the vegetables with the turmeric, pink salt, ground black pepper, and garlic powder.
4. Stir and cook the ingredients for 3 minutes.
5. After this, add shredded cauliflower and stir well.

6. Add almond milk. Stir the mixture again.
7. Close the lid and cook the meal for 6 minutes over the medium-high heat.
8. When the time is over – stir the meal carefully with the help of a spatula.

Nutrition value/serving: calories 113, fat 7.3, fiber 4.3, carbs 11.2, protein 3.7

8. Baked Asparagus with Eggs

Preparation time: 10 minutes
Cooking time: 13 minutes
Servings: 2
Ingredients:
- 2 eggs
- 8 oz asparagus
- 1 garlic clove, diced
- 1 teaspoon salt
- 1 tablespoon butter
- 1 oz almonds, chopped
- 4 tablespoon waters
- ½ teaspoon dried rosemary
- 1 tablespoon chopped parsley

Directions:
1. Preheat the oven to 365F.
2. Chop the asparagus roughly and sprinkle it with salt and dried rosemary.
3. Put the chopped vegetables in the springform pan. Add butter and water.
4. Cook the asparagus in the preheated oven for 8 minutes.
5. Stir the vegetables every 4 minutes.
6. Then remove the vegetables from the oven.
7. Sprinkle them with diced garlic and almonds, stir.
8. After this, beat the eggs over asparagus and transfer back in the oven.
9. Cook the meal for 5 minutes more or until the eggs are firm.

Nutrition value/serving: calories 222, fat 17.4, fiber 4.4, carbs 8.6, protein 11.3

9. Broccoli Fritters

Preparation time: 10 minutes

Cooking time: 10 minutes

Servings: 4

Ingredients:

- 1-pound broccoli
- 1 teaspoon chili flakes
- 2 eggs, beaten
- 4 oz Parmesan, grated
- 2 tablespoon almond meal
- 4 tablespoon ground flax meal
- 3 tablespoon olive oil

Directions:

1. Chop broccoli roughly and put in the food processor.
2. Add chili flakes, beaten eggs, grated cheese, and almond flour.
3. Blend the mixture until you get a smooth batter.
4. After this, make the medium balls from the batter and coat them in the flax meal.
5. Preheat the skillet well and add olive oil.
6. Preheat it.
7. Cook the broccoli balls for 2 minutes from each side or until light brown.

Nutrition value/serving: calories 298, fat 23.1, fiber 5.3, carbs 11.4, protein 17.2

10. Green Beans Salad

Preparation time: 5 minutes

Cooking time: 15 minutes

Servings: 3

Ingredients:

- 1 cup green beans, chopped
- 6 oz cauliflower florets
- 1 cup of water
- 1 teaspoon salt
- 1 teaspoon dried oregano
- 1 cup lettuce, chopped
- 2 tablespoon canola oil
- 1 tablespoon mustard

Directions:

1. In the saucepan combine together green beans and broccoli florets.
2. Add salt, close the lid, and cook the vegetables for 10 minutes over the medium-high heat.
3. Meanwhile, mix up together dried oregano, 1 tablespoon canola oil, and mustard in the mixing bowl. Whisk the mixture.
4. Then preheat the skillet.
5. Strain the vegetables and transfer them in the preheated skillet.
6. Add remaining canola oil and roast for 2 minutes over the high heat.
7. Put the chopped lettuce in the salad bowl.
8. Add roasted vegetables and mustard mixture.
9. Shake gently.

Nutrition value/serving: calories 130, fat 10.6, fiber 3.6, carbs 7.8, protein 2.9

11. Risotto

Preparation time: 10 minutes

Cooking time: 25 minutes

Servings: 4

Ingredients:

- 1 teaspoon butter
- 8 oz cauliflower, riced
- 1 white onion, diced
- 1 teaspoon pink salt
- 1 teaspoon ground black pepper
- 1 garlic clove, crushed
- 5 oz cremini mushrooms, chopped
- 1 tablespoon olive oil
- ½ cup almond milk
- 5 oz firmed tofu
- ½ cup of water

Directions:

1. Pour butter and olive oil in the saucepan and preheat.
2. Add diced onion, ground black pepper, salt, and crushed garlic.
3. Cook the spices for 2-3 minutes over the medium-high heat.
4. Add chopped mushrooms, onion, and water.
5. Close the lid and simmer the vegetables for 10 minutes.
6. Then add rice cauliflower and almond milk. Stir gently and cook for 5 minutes more.
7. Meanwhile, crumble tofu.
8. Add tofu in the meal and stir well. Cook it for 5 minutes more.

Nutrition value/serving: calories 169, fat 13.2, fiber 3.4, carbs 9.9, protein 6

RECIPES FOR DINNER

12. Parmesan Zucchini Fritters

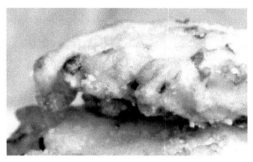

Preparation Time: 15 minutes

Cooking Time: 12-15 minutes

Serving: 9 zucchini fritters

Ingredients

- 3 medium zucchinis
- 2 teaspoons sea salt
- ½ cup superfine blanched almond flour
- ¼ cup grated Parmesan cheese
- 1 large egg
- ¼ teaspoon lemon pepper
- ½ teaspoon baking powder
- ½ teaspoon smoked paprika
- ½ teaspoon Italian seasoning
- ½ teaspoon garlic powder
- 2 green onions, finely sliced
- Avocado oil or olive oil

Directions:

    a. Grate the zucchini on a box grater or in a food processor. Put the zucchini in a colander and sprinkle with the sea salt. Mix the zucchini gently to distribute the salt and leave for 10 minutes.

2. After 10 minutes, use a good quality paper towel or clean dish towel and squeeze the excess water from the zucchini until the zucchini is dry.

3. Place it into a mixing bowl. Add egg, almond flour, ¼ cup grated Parmesan cheese, green onions and seasonings then mix until combined. If your batter still seems quite 'wet', add a little more flour.

4. Place a large cast iron or non-stick skillet over medium heat and add the oil, about 2 tablespoons.

5. Once the oil is heated, drop 1½ tablespoon-sized portions into the pan then gently press the batter to flatten. Fry for about 2-4 minutes on each side, until golden brown.

6. Drain the zucchini fritters on a paper towel before serving.

7. Repeat with remaining batter.

8. Serve warm or room temperature.

Nutritional Facts Per serving (1 zucchini fritter) ǀ Calories: 68 ǀ Total Fats: 5g ǀ Carbohydrates: 3g ǀ Fiber: 1g ǀ Protein: 4g ǀ Sugars: 1g

13. Bok Choy and Mushroom Stir-Fry

Preparation Time: 10 minutes

Cooking Time: 10 minutes

Serving: 4

Ingredients

- 1 pound baby bok choy
- 4 teaspoons vegetable oil
- 2 garlic cloves, chopped
- 1 teaspoon minced fresh ginger
- 5 ounces small fresh mushrooms, such as shiitake, button, beech, or enoki (cut into clumps), rinsed, tough parts of stems trimmed
- 2 tablespoons dry sherry
- 1 tablespoon soy sauce
- 2 teaspoons toasted sesame oil
- 1/8 teaspoon each kosher salt and pepper

Directions

1. Trim bases of bok choy and separate outer leaves from stalks, leaving the smallest inner leaves attached.
2. Rinse bok choy then dry with paper towels or a salad spinner.
3. Heat a wok or large frying pan (not nonstick) over medium-high heat. Once hot, add vegetable oil, chopped garlic, and ginger and stir once then immediately add mushrooms and cook, stirring constantly, until they just begin to brown, 1 to 2 minutes.
4. Add dry sherry and cook 30 seconds.
5. Add bok choy leaves and stalks and cook, tossing with tongs, for 1-2 minutes or until wilted.
6. Pour in soy sauce and sesame oil.
7. Season with salt and pepper.

8. Cook, tossing often, until bok choy is tender-crisp, an additional 1-2 minutes.

Nutritional Facts Per serving (¼ of recipe) Calories: 101 Total Fats: 7.3g Carbohydrates: 6.4g Fiber: 2g Protein: 2.7g

14. Green Beans in Tomato Sauce

Preparation Time: 10 minutes

Cooking Time: 25 minutes

Serving: 4

Ingredients

- 1-pound green beans (approximately)
- 2 tablespoons extra virgin olive oil
- 1 small-medium onion, finely chopped
- Pinch crushed red pepper flakes, optional
- 2 cloves garlic, minced
- 5 medium fresh tomatoes, blanched and chopped or 1 can (14 ounces) Italian peeled and crushed tomatoes
- 1-2 sprigs of fresh basil, chopped
- 1-2 sprigs of fresh parsley, chopped
- Salt and pepper to taste

Directions

1. Wash and trim the ends of the green beans. Set aside.
2. Place a large skillet over medium heat and add olive oil. Once the oil is heated, add the chopped onion and sauté, stirring occasionally, for about 4-5 minutes or until the onion is translucent.
3. Stir in garlic and red pepper flakes; cook and stir 1 minute.
4. Add the tomatoes.
5. Increase heat and bring mixture to boil then reduce heat and simmer 9-10 minutes or until the sauce starts to thicken.
6. In the meantime, bring a large pot of salted water to boil.
7. Add the green beans to the boiling water and cook, uncovered, until slightly tender but still crisp, about 5 minutes.
8. Drain beans in a colander and add to simmering tomatoes.

9. Simmer, uncovered, until beans become tender but still firm (not mushy), about 2-4 minutes. During the last minute of cooking, stir in basil and parsley.
10. Season with salt and pepper then taste and adjust seasoning as necessary.
11. Serve and enjoy!

Nutritional Facts Per serving (¼ of recipe) Calories: 131 Total Fats: 7g Carbohydrates: 15g Fiber: 5g Protein: 3g Sugar: 8g

15. Slow-Cooker Caponata

Preparation Time: 20 minutes
Cooking Time: 5 hours
Serving: 6 cups

Ingredients

- 2 medium eggplants, cut into ½-inch pieces
- 1 medium onion, chopped
- 1 can (14½ ounces) diced tomatoes, undrained
- 12 garlic cloves, sliced
- ½ cup dry red wine
- 3 tablespoons extra virgin olive oil
- 2 tablespoons red wine vinegar
- 4 teaspoons capers, undrained
- 5 bay leaves
- 1½ teaspoons salt
- ¼ teaspoon coarsely ground pepper
- Optional: toasted pine nuts

Directions

1. Add all ingredients, except pine nuts, in a 6-quart slow cooker. Do not stir.
2. Cook, covered, on high for 3 hours. Stir gently; replace cover. Cook on high until vegetables are tender, about 2 hours.
3. Allow to cool slightly. Remove and discard bay leaves
4. Transfer the caponata to a serving bowl and top with pine nuts.

Nutritional Facts Per serving (¼ cup) Calories: 34 Total Fats: 2g Carbohydrates: 4g Fiber: 2g Protein: 1g Sugar: 2g

16. Mushroom Cheese Empanadas

Preparation Time: 1 hour 10 minutes

Cooking Time: 15 minutes

Serving: 8

Ingredients

For the Dough:

- ¾ cup almond flour
- 6 tablespoons coconut flour
- 1 teaspoon xanthan gum
- ½ teaspoon salt
- ½ teaspoon garlic powder
- 1 teaspoon Italian seasoning
- 5 tablespoons butter
- 2 tablespoons cream cheese
- 2 eggs, separated (1 is for the egg wash)
- 1 teaspoon apple cider vinegar

For the Filling:

- 1 cup diced green onions
- 1 cup diced green peppers
- 2 tablespoons butter
- 1 cup diced mushrooms
- 1 cup mozzarella cheese

Directions

a. To make the dough: Measure the almond flour, coconut flour, garlic powder, xanthan gum, salt and Italian seasoning into a large bowl; whisk to aerate them.

2. With food processor: Add the mixed dry ingredients, cold butter, and cold cream cheese to your food processor then pulse several times to create a crumbly dough.

3. By hand: Add the cold cream cheese and cold butter to the flour mixture. Cut the butter and cheese into the dry ingredients, using your hands or your pastry blender.
4. Add one egg and apple cider vinegar and mix until a dough ball has formed. The dough will separate a bit, which is fine as it creates a flaky crust. Wrap dough in plastic wrap and chill in the fridge for 1 hour.
5. Remove dough from the fridge. Then place the dough between parchment paper and roll it sandwiched between those papers. For an empanada, you will want to get it thin but still be able to pick it up and fold.
6. Using a 4.5" round cookie cutter, cut out rounds and place them on a parchment-lined baking sheet. Transfer the baking sheet to the fridge to chill while preparing the filling.
7. To make the filling: Place a skillet over medium heat and add onions, peppers, butter and mushrooms. Sauté for 6-8 minutes then remove from the heat.
8. To assemble empanadas: Preheat oven to 375°F. Remove baking sheet of empanada dough circles from the fridge. Place about 1 tablespoon filling in the center of each round and top with cheese. Fold dough in half over filling. Use a fork to crimp edges together. Repeat with remaining filling and dough.
8. To cook empanadas: Whisk the remaining egg in a small bowl and brush the empanadas with egg wash. Bake for 15 minutes or until golden brown. Let cool a few minutes before serving.

Nutritional Facts Per serving (1 empanada) Calories: 192 Total Fats: 17g Carbohydrates: 6g Fiber: 4g Protein: 7g

RECIPES FOR VEGAN AND VEGETABLES

17. Grilled Portobello with Mashed Potatoes and Green Beans

Preparation time: 20 minutes

Cooking time: 40 minutes

Servings: 4

Ingredients

For the grilled portobellos

- 4 large portobello mushrooms
- 1 teaspoon olive oil
- Pinch sea salt

For the mashed potatoes

- 6 large potatoes, scrubbed or peeled, and chopped
- 3 to 4 garlic cloves, minced
- ½ teaspoon olive oil
- ½ cup non-dairy milk
- 2 tablespoons coconut oil (optional
- 2 tablespoons nutritional yeast (optional
- Pinch sea salt

For the green beans

- 2 cups green beans, cut into 1-inch pieces
- 2 to 3 teaspoons coconut oil
- Pinch sea salt
- 1 to 2 tablespoons nutritional yeast (optional

Directions

To Make the Grilled Portobellos

1. Preheat the grill to medium, or the oven to 350°F.

2. Take the stems out of the mushrooms.
3. Wipe the caps clean with a damp paper towel, then dry them. Spray the caps with a bit of olive oil, or put some oil in your hand and rub it over the mushrooms.
4. Rub the oil onto the top and bottom of each mushroom, then sprinkle them with a bit of salt on top and bottom.
5. Put them bottom side facing up on a baking sheet in the oven, or straight on the grill. They'll take about 30 minutes in the oven, or 20 minutes on the grill. Wait until they're soft and wrinkling around the edges. If you keep them bottom up, all the delicious mushroom juice will pool in the cap. Then at the very end, you can flip them over to drain the juice. If you like it, you can drizzle it over the mashed potatoes.
6. To Make the Mashed Potatoes
7. Boil the chopped potatoes in lightly salted water for about 20 minutes, until soft. While they're cooking, sauté the garlic in the olive oil, or bake them whole in a 350°F oven for 10 minutes, then squeeze out the flesh. Drain the potatoes, reserving about ½ cup water to mash them. In a large bowl, mash the potatoes with a little bit of the reserved water, the cooked garlic, milk, coconut oil (if using), nutritional yeast (if using), and salt to taste. Add more water, a little at a time, if needed, to get the texture you want. If you use an immersion blender or beater to purée them, you'll have some extra-creamy potatoes.

To Make the Green Bean
8. Heat a medium pot with a small amount of water to boil, then steam the green beans by either putting them directly in the pot or in a steaming basket.

9. Once they're slightly soft and vibrantly green, 7 to 8 minutes, take them off the heat and toss them with the oil, salt, and nutritional yeast (if using).

Nutrition: Calories: 263; Total fat: 7g; Carbs: 43g; Fiber: 7g; Protein: 10g

18. Tahini Broccoli Slaw

Preparation time: 15 minutes

Cooking time: 0 minutes

Servings: 4 to 6

Ingredients

- 1/4 cup tahini (sesame paste)
- 2 tablespoons white miso
- 1 tablespoon rice vinegar
- 1 tablespoon toasted sesame oil
- 2 teaspoons soy sauce
- 1 (12-ouncebag broccoli slaw
- 2 green onions, minced
- 1/4 cup toasted sesame seeds

Directions

1. In a large bowl, whisk together the tahini, miso, vinegar, oil, and soy sauce. Add the broccoli slaw, green onions, and sesame seeds and toss to coat.
2. Set aside for 20 minutes before serving.

Nutrition: Calories: 263; Total fat: 7g; Carbs: 43g; Fiber: 7g; Protein: 10g

19. Roasted Cauliflower Tacos

Preparation time: 10 minutes

Cooking time: 30 minutes

Servings: 8 tacos

Ingredients:

For the roasted cauliflower

- 1 head cauliflower, cut into bite-size pieces
- 1 tablespoon olive oil (optional
- 2 tablespoons whole-wheat flour
- 2 tablespoons nutritional yeast
- 1 to 2 teaspoons smoked paprika
- ½ to 1 teaspoon chili powder
- Pinch sea salt

For the tacos

- 2 cups shredded lettuce
- 2 cups cherry tomatoes, quartered
- 2 carrots, scrubbed or peeled, and grated
- ½ cup Fresh Mango Salsa
- ½ cup Guacamole
- 8 small whole-grain or corn tortillas
- 1 lime, cut into 8 wedges

Directions

To Make the Roasted Cauliflower

1. Preheat the oven to 350°F. Lightly grease a large rectangular baking sheet with olive oil, or line it with parchment paper. In a large bowl, toss the cauliflower pieces with oil (if using), or just rinse them so they're wet. The idea is to get the seasonings to stick. In a smaller bowl, mix together the flour, nutritional yeast, paprika, chili powder, and salt.

2. Add the seasonings to the cauliflower, and mix it around with your hands to thoroughly coat. Spread the cauliflower on the baking sheet, and roast for 20 to 30 minutes, or until softened.

To Make the Tacos.

1. Prep the veggies, salsa, and guacamole while the cauliflower is roasting. Once the cauliflower is cooked, heat the tortillas for just a few minutes in the oven or in a small skillet. Set everything out on the table, and assemble your tacos as you go. Give a squeeze of fresh lime just before eating.

Nutrition (1 taco): Calories: 198; Total fat: 6g; Carbs: 32g; Fiber: 6g; Protein: 7g

20. Creamy Mint-Lime

Spaghetti Squash
Preparation time: 10 minutes
Cooking time: 30 minutes
Servings: 3

Ingredients

For the dressing

- 3 tablespoons tahini
- Zest and juice of 1 small lime
- 2 tablespoons fresh mint, minced
- 1 small garlic clove, pressed
- 1 tablespoon nutritional yeast
- Pinch sea salt

For the spaghetti squash

- 1 spaghetti squash
- Pinch sea salt
- 1 cup cherry tomatoes, chopped
- 1 cup chopped bell pepper, any color
- Freshly ground black pepper

Directions

To Make the Dressing

1. Make the dressing by whisking together the tahini and lime juice until thick, stirring in water if you need it, until smooth, then add the rest of the ingredients. Or you can purée all the ingredients in a blender.

To Make the Spaghetti Squash.

2. Put a large pot of water on high and bring to a boil. Cut the squash in half and scoop out the seeds. Put the squash halves in the pot with the salt, and boil for about 30 minutes. Carefully remove the squash from the pot and let it cool until you can safely handle it. Set half the squash aside for another

meal. Scoop out the squash from the skin, which stays hard like a shell, and break the strands apart. The flesh absorbs water while boiling, so set the "noodles" in a strainer for 10 minutes, tossing occasionally to drain. Transfer the cooked spaghetti squash to a large bowl and toss with the mint-lime dressing. Then top with the cherry tomatoes and bell pepper. Add an extra sprinkle of nutritional yeast and black pepper, if you wish.

Nutrition: Calories: 199; Total fat: 10g; Carbs: 27g; Fiber: 5g; Protein: 7g

21. Smoky Coleslaw

Preparation time: 10 minutes

Cooking time: 0 minutes

Servings: 6

Ingredients

- 1-pound shredded cabbage
- 1/3 cup vegan mayonnaise
- ¼ cup unseasoned rice vinegar
- 3 tablespoons plain vegan yogurt or plain soymilk
- 1 tablespoon vegan sugar
- ½ teaspoon salt
- ¼ teaspoon freshly ground black pepper
- ¼ teaspoon smoked paprika
- ¼ teaspoon chipotle powder

Directions

1. Put the shredded cabbage in a large bowl. In a medium bowl, whisk the mayonnaise, vinegar, yogurt, sugar, salt, pepper, paprika, and chipotle powder.
3. Pour over the cabbage, and mix with a spoon or spatula and until the cabbage shreds are coated. Divide the coleslaw evenly among 6 single-serving containers. Seal the lids.

Nutrition: Calories: 73; Fat: 4g; Protein: 1g; Carbohydrates: 8g; Fiber: 2g; Sugar: 5g; Sodium: 283mg

22. Simple Sesame Stir-Fry

Preparation time: 10 minutes
Cooking time: 20 minutes
Servings: 4

Ingredients

- 1 cup quinoa
- 2 cups water
- Pinch sea salt
- 1 head broccoli
- 1 to 2 teaspoons untoasted sesame oil, or olive oil
- 1 cup snow peas, or snap peas, ends trimmed and cut in half
- 1 cup frozen shelled edamame beans, or peas
- 2 cups chopped Swiss chard, or other large-leafed green
- 2 scallions, chopped
- 2 tablespoons water
- 1 teaspoon toasted sesame oil
- 1 tablespoon tamari, or soy sauce
- 2 tablespoons sesame seeds

Directions

1. Put the quinoa, water, and sea salt in a medium pot, bring it to a boil for a minute, then turn to low and simmer, covered, for 20 minutes. The quinoa is fully cooked when you see the swirl of the grains with a translucent center, and it is fluffy. Do not stir the quinoa while it is cooking.

2. Meanwhile, cut the broccoli into bite-size florets, cutting and pulling apart from the stem. Also chop the stem into bite-size pieces. Heat a large skillet to high, and sauté the broccoli in the untoasted sesame oil, with a pinch of salt to help it soften. Keep this moving continuously, so that it doesn't burn, and add an extra drizzle of oil if needed as you add the rest of the vegetables. Add the snow peas next, continuing to stir. Add

the edamame until they thaw. Add the Swiss chard and scallions at the same time, tossing for only a minute to wilt. Then add 2 tablespoons of water to the hot skillet so that it sizzles and finishes the vegetables with a quick steam.

4. Dress with the toasted sesame oil and tamari, and toss one last time. Remove from the heat immediately. Serve a scoop of cooked quinoa, topped with stir-fry and sprinkled with some sesame seeds, and an extra drizzle of tamari and/or toasted sesame oil if you like.

Nutrition: Calories: 334; Total fat: 13g; Carbs: 42g; Fiber: 9g; Protein: 17g

SIDES DISH

23. Mashed Cauliflower

Preparation time: 10 minutes

Cooking time: 15 minutes

Servings: 4

Ingredients:

- 2 teaspoon minced garlic
- 10 oz cauliflower
- 1 teaspoon lemon juice
- 3 tablespoon almond milk
- 1 teaspoon salt
- ½ teaspoon chili flakes
- 2 cups of water

Directions:

1. Pour water in the saucepan and add cauliflower.
2. Close the lid and boil it for 15 minutes or until the vegetable is soft.
3. Then strain the cauliflower and transfer it in the blender.
4. Add minced garlic, almond milk, lemon juice, salt, and chili flakes.
5. Blend the vegetable until smooth and soft.
6. Transfer the cooked mashed cauliflower in the serving bowls.

Nutrition value/serving: calories 46, fat 2.8, fiber 2.1, carbs 4.9, protein 1.8

24. Fragrant Cauliflower Steaks

Preparation time: 10 minutes

Cooking time: 10 minutes

Servings: 6

Ingredients:

- 2-pound cauliflower head
- 1 teaspoon Taco seasoning
- 1 teaspoon ground thyme
- 1 tablespoon butter
- 4 oz Parmesan, grated

Directions:

1. Preheat the grill to 365F.
2. Meanwhile, slice the cauliflower head into steaks.
3. Rub every cauliflower steak with Taco seasoning and ground thyme.
4. Place the steaks on the grill and grill for 2 minutes from each side.
5. After this, rub the cauliflower with butter and cook for 1 minute more from each side.
6. Then sprinkle the cauliflower steaks with grated cheese and cook for 3 minutes only on one side.

Nutrition value/serving: calories 118, fat 6.1, fiber 3.8, carbs 9.1, protein 9.1

25. Fried Cheese

Preparation time: 10 minutes

Cooking time: 5 minutes

Servings: 6

Ingredients:

- 1-pound goat cheese log
- 1/3 cup almond flour
- 1 egg, whisked
- 1 teaspoon chili pepper
- ½ teaspoon garlic powder
- 1 tablespoon olive oil

Directions:

1. Cut the goat cheese into medium pieces.
2. Then mix up together almond flour, chili pepper, and garlic powder. Stir it.
3. Dip the goat cheese pieces in the whisked egg.
4. Then coat them in the almond flour mixture.
5. Preheat the skillet and pour olive oil inside.
6. When the olive oil is hot, place the goat cheese inside and cook for 30 seconds from each side.
7. Serve the cooked side dish hot.

Nutrition value/serving: calories 362, fat 28.4, fiber 0.2, carbs 2.3, protein 24.4

26. Cabbage Salad

Preparation time: 8 minutes

Cooking time: 5 minutes

Servings: 2

Ingredients:

- 8 oz white cabbage, shredded
- ½ avocado, peeled
- 2 tablespoons lemon juice
- 1 teaspoon avocado oil
- ¼ cup spinach, chopped
- 3 tablespoon waters

Directions:

1. Place avocado, lemon juice, spinach, avocado oil, and water in the blender.
2. Blend the mixture until smooth.
3. Place the cabbage in the salad bowl.
4. Pour the green mixture over the cabbage.
5. Mix up the salad well and let it marinate for at least 5 minutes.

Nutrition value/serving: calories 156, fat 12.4, fiber 6.4, carbs 11.4, protein 2.6

27. Hummus

Preparation time: 10 minutes

Cooking time: 15 minutes

Servings: 6

Ingredients:

- 2-pound cauliflower head
- 1 teaspoon salt
- 1 teaspoon garlic powder
- 1 teaspoon chili flakes
- 3 tablespoon olive oil
- 1 tablespoon tahini paste
- 1 cup of water

Directions:

1. Boil cauliflower head in 1 cup of water for 15 minutes or until tender.
2. Meanwhile, mix up together salt, garlic powder, chili flakes, olive oil, and tahini paste.
3. Strain the cauliflower. Leave 5 tablespoons of cauliflower water.
4. Blend the vegetable until you get a mashed mixture.
5. Add 5 tablespoons of remaining cauliflower water and tahini paste mixture.
6. Blend the hummus for 2 minutes more.
7. Transfer it in the bowl.

Nutrition value/serving: calories 114, fat 8.5, fiber 4.1, carbs 8.9, protein 3.5

RECIPES FOR PASTA

28. Zucchini Vegan Bacon Lasagna

Preparation Time: 15 minutes
Cooking Time: 40 minutes
Serving: 4
Ingredients:

- 4 large yellow zucchinis
- Salt and black pepper to taste
- 1 tbsp lard
- ½ lb. vegan bacon
- 1 tsp garlic powder
- 1 tsp onion powder
- 2 tbsp coconut flour
- 1 ½ cup grated mozzarella cheese
- 1/3 cup cheddar cheese
- 2 cups crumbled ricotta cheese
- 1 large egg
- 2 cups unsweetened marinara sauce
- 1 tbsp Italian herb seasoning
- ¼ tsp red chili flakes
- ¼ cup fresh basil leaves

Directions:

1. Preheat the oven to 375 F and grease a 9 x 9-inch baking dish with cooking spray. Set aside.
2. Slice the zucchini into ¼ -inch strips, arrange on a flat surface and sprinkle generously with salt. Set aside to release liquid for 5 to 10 minutes. Pat dry with a paper towel and set aside.

3. Melt the lard in a large skillet over medium heat and add the vegan bacon. Cook until browned, 10 minutes. Set aside to cool.

4. In a medium bowl, evenly combine the garlic powder, onion powder, coconut flour, salt, black pepper, mozzarella cheese, half of the cheddar cheese, ricotta cheese, and egg. Set aside.

5. Add the Italian herb seasoning and red chili flakes to the marinara sauce and mix. Set aside.

6. Make a single layer of the zucchini in the baking dish; spread a quarter of the egg mixture on top, and a quarter of the marinara sauce. Repeat the layering process and sprinkle the top with the remaining cheddar cheese.

7. Bake in the oven for 30 minutes or until golden brown on top.

8. Remove the dish from the oven, allow cooling for 5 to 10 minutes, garnish with the basil leaves, slice and serve.

Nutrition: Calories:417, Total Fat: 36.4g, Saturated Fat: 15.9g, Total Carbs: 4g, Dietary Fiber:0g, Sugar: 1g, Protein20: g, Sodium: 525mg

29. Parsley-Lime Pasta

Preparation Time: 20 minutes
Cooking Time: 15 minutes
Serving: 4
Ingredients:
- 2 tbsp butter
- 1 lb. tempeh, chopped
- 4 garlic cloves, minced
- 1 pinch red chili flakes
- ¼ cup white wine
- 1 lime, zested and juiced
- 3 medium zucchinis, spiralized
- Salt and black pepper to taste
- 2 tbsp chopped parsley
- 1 cup grated parmesan cheese for topping

Directions:
1. Melt the butter in a large skillet and cook in the tempeh until golden brown.
2. Flip and stir in the garlic and red chili flakes. Cook further for 1 minute; transfer to a plate and set aside.
3. Pour the wine and lime juice into the skillet, and cook until reduced by a quarter. Meanwhile, stir to deglaze the bottom of the pot.
4. Mix in the zucchinis, lime zest, tempeh and parsley. Season with salt and black pepper, and toss everything well. Cook until the zucchinis are slightly tender for 2 minutes.
5. Dish the food onto serving plates and top generously with the parmesan cheese.

Nutrition: Calories: 326, Total Fat: 24.9g, Saturated Fat:12.9 g, Total Carbs: 6 g, Dietary Fiber:1g, Sugar: 4g, Protein: 20g, Sodium: 568mg

30. Creamy Garlic Mushrooms with Angel Hair Shirataki

Preparation Time: 25 minutes

Cooking Time: 15 minutes

Cooking Time:

Serving: 4

Ingredients:

For the mushroom sauce:

- 1 tbsp olive oil
- 1 lb. chopped mushrooms
- Salt and black pepper to taste
- 2 tbsp unsalted butter
- 6 garlic cloves, minced
- ½ cup dry white wine
- 1 ½ cups coconut cream
- ½ cup grated parmesan cheese
- 2 tbsp chopped fresh parsley
- For the angel hair shirataki:
- 2 (8 oz) packs angel hair shirataki noodles
- Salt to season

Directions:

For the mushroom sauce:

1. Heat the olive oil in a large skillet, season the mushroom with salt and black pepper, and cook in the oil until softened, 5 minutes. Transfer to a plate and set aside.
2. Melt the butter in the skillet and sauté the garlic until fragrant. Stir in the white wine and cook until reduced by half, meanwhile, scraping the bottom of the pan to deglaze.
3. Reduce the heat to low and stir in the coconut cream. Allow simmering for 1 minute and stir in the parmesan cheese to melt.

4. Return the mushroom to the sauce and sprinkle the parsley on top. Adjust the taste with salt and black pepper, if needed.

For the angel hair shirataki:

1. Bring 2 cups of water to a boil in a medium pot over medium heat.
2. Strain the shirataki pasta through a colander and rinse very well under hot running water.
3. Allow proper draining and pour the shirataki pasta into the boiling water. Cook for 3 minutes and strain again.
4. Place a dry skillet over medium heat and stir-fry the shirataki pasta until visibly dry and makes a squeaky sound when stirred, 1 to 2 minutes.
5. Season with salt and plate.
6. Top the shirataki pasta with the mushroom sauce and serve warm.

Nutrition: Calories:89, Total Fat:6.4 g, Saturated Fat:1.5 g, Total Carbs: 2g, Dietary Fiber:0g, Sugar:1g, Protein:6 g, Sodium: 406mg

31. Coconut Tofu Zucchini Bake

Preparation Time: 40 minutes
Cooking Time: 20 minutes
Serving: 4

Ingredients:
- 1 tbsp butter
- 1 cup green beans, chopped
- 1 bunch asparagus, trimmed and cut into 1-inch pieces
- 2 tbsp arrowroot starch
- 2 cups coconut milk
- 4 medium zucchinis, spiralized
- 1 cup grated parmesan cheese
- 1 (15 oz) firm tofu, pressed and sliced
- Salt and black pepper to taste

Directions:
1. Preheat the oven to 380 F.
2. Melt the butter in a medium skillet and sauté the green beans and asparagus until softened, about 5 minutes. Set aside.
3. In a medium saucepan, mix the arrowroot starch with the coconut milk. Bring to a boil over medium heat with frequent stirring until thickened, 3 minutes. Stir in half of the parmesan cheese until melted.
4. Mix in the green beans, asparagus, zucchinis and tofu. Season with salt and black pepper.
5. Transfer the mixture to a baking dish and cover the top with the remaining parmesan cheese.
6. Bake in the oven until the cheese melts and golden on top, 20 minutes.
7. Remove the food from the oven and serve warm.

Nutrition: Calories: 492, Total Fat:26.8 g, Saturated Fat: 12.6g, Total Carbs: 14g, Dietary Fiber:4g, Sugar: 8g, Protein: 50g, Sodium: 1668mg

32. Creamy Seitan Shirataki Fettucine

Preparation Time: 35 minutes

Cooking Time: 30 minutes

Serving: 4

Ingredients:

For the shirataki fettuccine:

- 2 (8 oz) packs shirataki fettuccine
- For the creamy seitan sauce:
- 5 tbsp butter
- 4 seitan slabs, cut into 2-inch cubes
- Salt and black pepper to taste
- 3 garlic cloves, minced
- 1 ¼ cups coconut cream
- ½ cup dry white wine
- 1 tsp grated lemon zest
- 1 cup baby spinach
- Lemon wedges for garnishing

Directions:

For the shirataki fettuccine:

1. Boil 2 cups of water in a medium pot over medium heat.
2. Strain the shirataki pasta through a colander and rinse very well under hot running water.
3. Allow proper draining and pour the shirataki pasta into the boiling water. Cook for 3 minutes and strain again.
4. Place a dry skillet over medium heat and stir-fry the shirataki pasta until visibly dry, and makes a squeaky sound when stirred, 1 to 2 minutes. Take off the heat and set aside.

For the seitan sauce:

5. Melt half of the butter in a large skillet; season the seitan with salt, black pepper, and cook in the butter until golden brown

on all sides and flaky within, 8 minutes. Transfer to a plate and set aside.

6. Add the remaining butter to the skillet to melt and stir in the garlic. Cook until fragrant, 1 minute.
7. Mix in the coconut cream, white wine, lemon zest, salt, and black pepper. Allow boiling over low heat until the sauce thickens, 5 minutes.
8. Stir in the spinach, allow wilting for 2 minutes and stir in the shirataki fettuccine and seitan until well-coated in the sauce. Adjust the taste with salt and black pepper.
9. Dish the food and garnish with the lemon wedges. Serve warm.

Nutrition: Calories: 720, Total Fat: 56.5g, Saturated Fat: 27.2g, Total Carbs: 17 g, Dietary Fiber:3g, Sugar: 7g, Protein: 37g, Sodium:1764 mg

RECIPES FOR SNACKS

33. Nori Snack Rolls

Preparation Time: 5 Minutes

Cooking Time: 10 Minutes

Servings: 4

Ingredients

- 2 tablespoons almond, cashew, peanut, or another nut butter
- 2 tablespoons tamari, or soy sauce
- 4 standard nori sheets
- 1 mushroom, sliced
- 1 tablespoon pickled ginger
- ½ cup grated carrots

Directions

1. Preheat the oven to 350°F.
2. Mix together the nut butter and tamari until smooth and very thick. Lay out a nori sheet, rough side up, the long way.
3. Spread a thin line of the tamari mixture on the far end of the nori sheet, from side to side. Lay the mushroom slices, ginger, and carrots in a line at the other end (the end closest to you).
4. Fold the vegetables inside the nori, rolling toward the tahini mixture, which will seal the roll. Repeat to make 4 rolls.
5. Put on a baking sheet and bake for 8 to 10 minutes, or until the rolls are slightly browned and crispy at the ends. Let the rolls cool for a few minutes, then slice each roll into 3 smaller pieces.

Nutrition: Calories: 79 Cal Fat: 5 g Carbs: 6 g Fiber: 2 g Protein: 4 g

34. Risotto Bites

Preparation Time: 15 Minutes

Cooking Time: 20 Minutes

Servings: 12

Ingredients

- ½ cup panko bread crumbs
- 1 teaspoon paprika
- 1 teaspoon chipotle powder or ground cayenne pepper
- 1½ cups cold Green Pea Risotto
- Nonstick cooking spray

Directions

1. Preheat the oven to 425ºF.
2. Line a baking sheet with parchment paper.
3. On a large plate, combine the panko, paprika, and chipotle powder. Set aside.
4. Roll 2 tablespoons of the risotto into a ball.
5. Gently roll in the bread crumbs, and place on the prepared baking sheet. Repeat to make a total of 12 balls.
6. Spritz the tops of the risotto bites with nonstick cooking spray and bake for 15 to 20 minutes, until they begin to brown. Cool completely before storing in a large airtight container in a single layer (add a piece of parchment paper for a second layer or in a plastic freezer bag.

Nutrition: Calories: 100 Cal Fat: 2 g Protein: 6 g Carbs: 17 g Fiber: 5 g

35. Jicama and Guacamole

Preparation Time: 15 Minutes

Cooking Time: 0

Servings: 4

Ingredients

- juice of 1 lime, or 1 tablespoon prepared lime juice
- 2 avocados, peeled, pits removed, and cut into cubes
- ½ teaspoon sea salt
- ½ red onion, minced
- 1 garlic clove, minced
- ¼ cup chopped cilantro (optional
- 1 jicama bulb, peeled and cut into matchsticks

Directions

1. In a medium bowl, squeeze the lime juice over the top of the avocado and sprinkle with salt.
2. Lightly mash the avocado with a fork. Stir in the onion, garlic, and cilantro, if using.
3. Serve with slices of jicama to dip in guacamole.
4. To store, place plastic wrap over the bowl of guacamole and refrigerate. The guacamole will keep for about 2 days.

Nutrition: Calories: 130 Cal Fat: 2 g Protein: 5 g Carbs: 13 g Fiber: 5 g

36. Curried Tofu "Egg Salad" Pitas

Preparation Time: 15 Minutes

Cooking Time: 0 Minutes

Servings: 4 Sandwiches

Ingredients

- 1-pound extra-firm tofu, drained and patted dry
- 1/2 cup vegan mayonnaise, homemade or store-bought
- 1/4 cup chopped mango chutney, homemade or store-bought
- 2 teaspoons Dijon mustard
- 1 tablespoon hot or mild curry powder
- 1 teaspoon salt
- 1/8 teaspoon ground cayenne
- 3/4 cup shredded carrots
- 2 celery ribs, minced
- 1/4 cup minced red onion
- 8 small Boston or other soft lettuce leaves
- 4 (7-inchwhole wheat pita breads, halved

Directions

1. Crumble the tofu and place it in a large bowl. Add the mayonnaise, chutney, mustard, curry powder, salt, and cayenne, and stir well until thoroughly mixed.
2. Add the carrots, celery, and onion and stir to combine. Refrigerate for 30 minutes to allow the flavors to blend.
3. Tuck a lettuce leaf inside each pita pocket, spoon some tofu mixture on top of the lettuce, and serve.

Nutrition: Calories: 200 Cal Fat: 3 g Protein: 9 g Carbs: 11 g Fiber: 8 g

37. Garden Patch Sandwiches on Multigrain Bread

Preparation Time: 15 Minutes

Cooking Time: 0 Minutes

Servings: 4 Sandwiches

Ingredients

- 1pound extra-firm tofu, drained and patted dry
- 1 medium red bell pepper, finely chopped
- 1 celery rib, finely chopped
- 3 green onions, minced
- 1/4 cup shelled sunflower seeds
- 1/2 cup vegan mayonnaise, homemade or store-bought
- 1/2 teaspoon salt
- 1/2 teaspoon celery salt
- 1/4 teaspoon freshly ground black pepper
- 8 slices whole grain bread
- 4 1/4-inchslices ripe tomato
- 4 lettuce leaves

Directions

1. Crumble the tofu and place it in a large bowl. Add the bell pepper, celery, green onions, and sunflower seeds. Stir in the mayonnaise, salt, celery salt, and pepper and mix until well combined.

2. Toast the bread, if desired. Spread the mixture evenly onto 4 slices of the bread. Top each with a tomato slice, lettuce leaf, and the remaining bread. Cut the sandwiches diagonally in half and serve.

Nutrition: Calories: 234 Cal Fat: 6 g Protein: 3 g Carbs: 12 g Fiber: 9 g

38. Garden Salad Wraps

Preparation Time: 15 Minutes
Cooking Time: 10 Minutes
Servings: 4 Wraps

Ingredients

- 6 tablespoons olive oil
- 1-pound extra-firm tofu, drained, patted dry, and cut into 1/2-inch strips
- 1 tablespoon soy sauce
- 1/4 cup apple cider vinegar
- 1 teaspoon yellow or spicy brown mustard
- 1/2 teaspoon salt
- 1/4 teaspoon freshly ground black pepper
- 3 cups shredded romaine lettuce
- 3 ripe Roma tomatoes, finely chopped
- 1 large carrot, shredded
- 1 medium English cucumber, peeled and chopped
- 1/3 cup minced red onion
- 1/4 cup sliced pitted green olives
- 4 (10-inchwhole-grain flour tortillas or lavash flatbread

Directions

1. In a large skillet, heat 2 tablespoons of the oil over medium heat.
2. Add the tofu and cook until golden brown, about 10 minutes.
3. Sprinkle with soy sauce and set aside to cool.
4. In a small bowl, combine the vinegar, mustard, salt, and pepper with the remaining 4 tablespoons oil, stirring to blend well. Set aside.
5. In a large bowl, combine the lettuce, tomatoes, carrot, cucumber, onion, and olives. Pour on the dressing and toss to coat.

6. To assemble wraps, place 1 tortilla on a work surface and spread with about one-quarter of the salad.
7. Place a few strips of tofu on the tortilla and roll up tightly. Slice in half

Nutrition: Calories: 200 Cal Fat: 5 g Protein: 6 g Carbs: 7 g Fiber: 7 g

RECIPES FOR SOUP AND STEW

39. Chickpea And Black Olive Stew

Preparation Time: 15-30 minutes

Cooking Time: 15 minutes

Servings: 4

Ingredients:

- 2 tbsp olive oil
- 2 cups chopped onion
- 2 garlic cloves, minced
- 2 carrots, peeled and cut into thick slices
- 1/3 cup white wine
- 3 cups cherry tomatoes
- 2/3 cup vegetable stock
- 1 1/3 cups canned chickpeas, drained and rinsed
- ½ cup pitted black olives
- 1 tbsp chopped fresh oregano

Directions:

1. Heat the olive oil in a medium pot and sauté the onion, garlic, and carrots until softened, 5 minutes.
2. Mix in the white wine, allow reduction by one-third, and mix in the tomatoes, and vegetable stock. Cover the lid and cook until the tomatoes break, soften, and the liquid reduces by half.
3. Stir in the chickpeas, olives, oregano and season with salt and black pepper. Cook for 3 minutes to warm the chickpeas.
4. Dish the stew and serve warm.

Nutrition: Calories 698 kcal Fats 51. 3 g Carbs 54. 1 g Protein 12. 1g

40. Lentil and Wild Rice Soup

Preparation Time: 10 minutes
Cooking Time: 40 minutes
Servings: 4

Ingredients:

- 1/2 cup cooked mixed beans
- 12 ounces cooked lentils
- 2 stalks of celery, sliced
- 1 1/2 cup mixed wild rice, cooked
- 1 large sweet potato, peeled, chopped
- 1/2 medium butternut, peeled, chopped
- 4 medium carrots, peeled, sliced
- 1 medium onion, peeled, diced
- 10 cherry tomatoes
- 1/2 red chili, deseeded, diced
- 1 ½ teaspoon minced garlic
- 1/2 teaspoon salt
- 2 teaspoons mixed dried herbs
- 1 teaspoon coconut oil
- 2 cups vegetable broth

Directions:

1. Take a large pot, place it over medium-high heat, add oil and when it melts, add onion and cook for 5 minutes.
2. Stir in garlic and chili, cook for 3 minutes, then add remaining vegetables, pour in the broth, stir and bring the mixture to a boil.
3. Switch heat to medium-low heat, cook the soup for 20 minutes, then stir in remaining ingredients and continue cooking for 10 minutes until soup has reached the desired thickness.
4. Serve straight away.

Nutrition: Calories: 331 Cal Fat: 2 g Carbs: 54 g Protein: 13 g Fiber: 12 g

41. Garlic and White Bean Soup

Preparation Time: 10 minutes

Cooking Time: 10 minutes

Servings: 4

Ingredients:

- 45 ounces cooked cannellini beans
- 1/4 teaspoon dried thyme
- 2 teaspoons minced garlic
- 1/8 teaspoon crushed red pepper
- 1/2 teaspoon dried rosemary
- 1/8 teaspoon ground black pepper
- 2 tablespoons olive oil
- 4 cups vegetable broth

Directions:

1. Place one-third of white beans in a food processor, then pour in 2 cups of broth and pulse for 2 minutes until smooth.
2. Place a pot over medium heat, add oil and when hot, add garlic and cook for 1 minute until fragrant. Add pureed beans into the pan along with remaining beans, sprinkle with spices and herbs, pour in the broth, stir until combined, and bring the mixture to boil over medium-high heat. Switch heat to medium-low level, simmer the beans for 15 minutes, and then mash them with a fork. Taste the soup to adjust seasoning and then serve.

Nutrition: Calories: 222 Cal Fat: 7 g Carbs: 13 g Protein: 11. 2 g Fiber: 9. 1 g

42. Vegetarian Irish Stew

Preparation Time: 5 minutes
Cooking Time: 38 minutes
Servings: 6
Ingredients:
- 1 cup textured vegetable protein, chunks
- ½ cup split red lentils
- 2 medium onions, peeled, sliced
- 1 cup sliced parsnip
- 2 cups sliced mushrooms
- 1 cup diced celery,
- 1/4 cup flour
- 4 cups vegetable stock
- 1 cup rutabaga
- 1 bay leaf
- ½ cup fresh parsley
- 1 teaspoon sugar
- ¼ teaspoon ground black pepper
- 1/4 cup soy sauce
- ¼ teaspoon thyme
- 2 teaspoons marmite
- ¼ teaspoon rosemary
- 2/3 teaspoon salt
- ¼ teaspoon marjoram

Directions:
1. Take a large soup pot, place it over medium heat, add oil and when it gets hot, add onions and cook for 5 minutes until softened.
2. Then switch heat to the low level, sprinkle with flour, stir well, add remaining ingredients, stir until combined, and simmer for 30 minutes until vegetables have cooked.

3. When done, season the stew with salt and black pepper and then serve.

Nutrition: Calories: 117.4 Cal Fat: 4 g Carbs: 22.8 g Protein: 6.5 g Fiber: 7.3 g

43. White Bean and Cabbage Stew

Preparation Time: 5 minutes
Cooking Time: 8 hours
Servings: 4
Ingredients:

- 3 cups cooked great northern beans
- 1.5 pounds potatoes, peeled, cut into large dice
- 1 large white onion, peeled, chopped
- ½ head of cabbage, chopped
- 3 ribs celery, chopped
- 4 medium carrots, peeled, sliced
- 14.5 ounces diced tomatoes
- 1/3 cup pearled barley
- 1 teaspoon minced garlic
- ½ teaspoon ground black pepper
- 1 bay leaf
- 1 teaspoon dried thyme
- ½ teaspoon crushed rosemary
- 1 teaspoon salt
- ½ teaspoon caraway seeds
- 1 tablespoon chopped parsley
- 8 cups vegetable broth

Directions:

1. Switch on the slow cooker, then add all the ingredients except for salt, parsley, tomatoes, and beans and stir until mixed.
2. Shut the slow cooker with a lid, and cook for 7 hours at a low heat setting until cooked.
3. Then stir in remaining ingredients, stir until combined, and continue cooking for 1 hour.
4. Serve straight away

Nutrition: Calories: 150 Cal Fat: 0.7 g Carbs: 27 g Protein: 7 g Fiber: 9.4 g

44. Black Bean Taco Salad Bowl

Preparation time: 15 minutes

Cooking time: 5 minutes

Servings: 3

Ingredients

For the black bean salad

- 1 (14-ouncecan black beans, drained and rinsed, or 1½ cups cooked
- 1 cup corn kernels, fresh and blanched, or frozen and thawed
- ¼ cup fresh cilantro, or parsley, chopped
- Zest and juice of 1 lime
- 1 to 2 teaspoons chili powder
- Pinch sea salt
- 1½ cups cherry tomatoes, halved
- 1 red bell pepper, seeded and chopped
- 2 scallions, chopped
- For 1 serving of tortilla chips
- 1 large whole-grain tortilla or wrap
- 1 teaspoon olive oil
- Pinch sea salt
- Pinch freshly ground black pepper
- Pinch dried oregano

Pinch chili powder

- For 1 bowl
- 1 cup fresh greens (lettuce, spinach, or whatever you like
- ¾ cup cooked quinoa, or brown rice, millet, or other whole grain

- ¼ cup chopped avocado, or Guacamole
- ¼ cup Fresh Mango Salsa

Directions

1. To make the black bean salad
2. Toss all the ingredients together in a large bowl.
3. To make the tortilla chips
4. Brush the tortilla with olive oil, then sprinkle with salt, pepper, oregano, chili powder, and any other seasonings you like. Slice it into eighths like a pizza.
5. Transfer the tortilla pieces to a small baking sheet lined with parchment paper and put in the oven or toaster oven to toast or broil for 3 to 5 minutes, until browned. Keep an eye on them, as they can go from just barely done to burned very quickly.
6. To make the bowl
7. Lay the greens in the bowl, top with the cooked quinoa, 1/3 of the black bean salad, the avocado, and salsa.

Nutrition: Calories: 589; Total fat: 14g; Carbs: 101g; Fiber: 20g; Protein: 21g

45. Warm Vegetable "Salad"

Preparation time: 10 minutes
Cooking time: 15 minutes
Servings: 4

Ingredients

- Salt for salting water, plus ½ teaspoon (optional
- 4 red potatoes, quartered
- 1-pound carrots, sliced into ¼-inch-thick rounds
- 1 tablespoon extra-virgin olive oil (optional
- 2 tablespoons lime juice
- 2 teaspoons dried dill
- ¼ teaspoon freshly ground black pepper
- 1 cup Cashew Cream or Parm-y Kale Pesto

Directions

1. In a large pot, bring salted water to a boil. Add the potatoes and cook for 8 minutes. Add the carrots and continue to boil for another 8 minutes, until both the potatoes and carrots are crisp tender. Drain and return to the pot. Add the olive oil (if using), lime juice, dill, remaining ½ teaspoon of salt (if using), and pepper, and stir to coat well.

2. Divide the vegetables evenly among 4 single-compartment storage containers or wide-mouth pint glass jars, and spoon ¼ cup of cream or pesto over the vegetables in each. Let cool before sealing the lids.

Nutrition: Calories: 393; Fat: 15g; Protein: 10g; Carbohydrates: 52g; Fiber: 9g; Sugar: 8g; Sodium: 343mg

46. Caramelized Onion and Beet Salad

Preparation time: 10 minutes

Cooking time: 40 minutes

Servings: 4

Ingredients

- 3 medium golden beets
- 2 cups sliced sweet or Vidalia onions
- 1 teaspoon extra-virgin olive oil or no-beef broth
- Pinch baking soda
- ¼ to ½ teaspoon salt, to taste
- 2 tablespoons unseasoned rice vinegar, white wine vinegar, or balsamic vinegar

Directions

1. Cut the greens off the beets, and scrub the beets.
2. In a large pot, place a steamer basket and fill the pot with 2 inches of water.
3. Add the beets, bring to a boil, then reduce the heat to medium, cover, and steam for about 35 minutes, until you can easily pierce the middle of the beets with a knife.
4. Meanwhile, in a large, dry skillet over medium heat, sauté the onions for 5 minutes, stirring frequently.
5. Add the olive oil and baking soda, and continuing cooking for 5 more minutes, stirring frequently. Stir in the salt to taste before removing from the heat. Transfer to a large bowl and set aside.
6. When the beets have cooked through, drain and cool until easy to handle. Rub the beets in a paper towel to easily remove the skins. Cut into wedges, and transfer to the bowl with the onions. Drizzle the vinegar over everything and toss well.
7. Divide the beets evenly among 4 wide-mouth jars or storage containers. Let cool before sealing the lids.

Nutrition: Calories: 104; Fat: 2g; Protein: 3g; Carbohydrates: 20g; Fiber: 4g; Sugar: 14g; Sodium: 303mg

47. Warm Lentil Salad with Red Wine Vinaigrette

Preparation time: 10 minutes

Cooking time: 50 minutes

Servings: 4

Ingredients

- 1 teaspoon olive oil plus ¼ cup, divided, or 1 tablespoon vegetable broth or water
- 1 small onion, diced
- 1 garlic clove, minced
- 1 carrot, diced
- 1 cup lentils
- 1 tablespoon dried basil
- 1 tablespoon dried oregano
- 1 tablespoon red wine or balsamic vinegar (optional
- 2 cups water
- ¼ cup red wine vinegar or balsamic vinegar
- 1 teaspoon sea salt
- 2 cups chopped Swiss chard
- 2 cups torn red leaf lettuce
- 4 tablespoons Cheesy Sprinkle

Directions

1. Heat 1 teaspoon of the oil in a large pot on medium heat, then sauté the onion and garlic until they are translucent, about 5 minutes.

2. Add the carrot and sauté until it is slightly cooked, about 3 minutes. Stir in the lentils, basil, and oregano, then add the wine or balsamic vinegar (if using).

3. Pour the water into the pot and turn the heat up to high to bring to a boil.

4. Turn the heat down to a simmer and let the lentils cook, uncovered, 20 to 30 minutes, until they are soft but not falling apart.

5. While the lentils are cooking, whisk together the red wine vinegar, olive oil, and salt in a small bowl and set aside. Once the lentils have cooked, drain any excess liquid and stir in most of the red wine vinegar dressing. Set a little bit of dressing aside. Add the Swiss chard to the pot and stir it into the lentils. Leave the heat on low and cook, stirring, for at least 10 minutes. Toss the lettuce with the remaining dressing. Place some lettuce on a plate, and top with the lentil mixture. Finish the plate off with a little Cheesy Sprinkle and enjoy.

Nutrition Calories: 387; Total fat: 17g; Carbs: 42g; Fiber: 19g; Protein: 18g

48. Not-Tuna Salad

Preparation time: 5 minutes

Cooking time: 0 minutes

Servings: 4

Ingredients

- 1 (15.5-ouncecan chickpeas, drained and rinsed
- 1 (14-ouncecan hearts of palm, drained and chopped
- ½ cup chopped yellow or white onion
- ½ cup diced celery
- ¼ cup vegan mayonnaise, plus more if needed
- ½ teaspoon salt
- ¼ teaspoon freshly ground black pepper

Directions

1. In a medium bowl, use a potato masher or fork to roughly mash the chickpeas until chunky and "shredded." Add the hearts of palm, onion, celery, vegan mayonnaise, salt, and pepper.
2. Combine and add more mayonnaise, if necessary, for a creamy texture. Into each of 4 single-serving containers, place ¾ cup of salad. Seal the lids.

Nutrition: Calories: 214; Fat: 6g; Protein: 9g; Carbohydrates: 35g; Fiber: 8g; Sugar: 1g; Sodium: 765mg

49. Bounty Bars

Preparation Time: 10 minutes + about 1 hour Cooling Time

Cooking Time: 0 minutes

Serving: 20 bars

Ingredients

- 1 cup coconut butter, melted
- ¼ cup monk fruit sweetened maple syrup
- 2½ cups unsweetened shredded coconut
- 2 cups stevia sweetened chocolate chips

Directions

1. In a small bowl, microwave coconut butter and maple syrup until smooth and creamy. Stir in coconut flakes.
2. Line an 8×8-inch pan with parchment paper, add the coconut mixture, and press firmly in place. Refrigerate for 30 minutes or until firm.
3. Cut into 20 bars and set aside.
4. In a microwave safe bowl, add the chocolate chips and melt it in the microwave for 1 minute.
5. With a fork, dip each bar in chocolate until it is well-coated.
6. Refrigerate until firm.
7. Store in an airtight container in the fridge.

Nutrition: Per serving (1 bar) | Calories: 111 | Total Fats: 11g | Carbohydrates: 5g | Fiber: 3g | Protein: 1g

50. Lemon Cookies

Preparation Time: 10 minutes
Cooking Time: 8 minutes
Serving: 9 cookies

Ingredients

- ½ cup unsalted grass-fed butter, softened to room temperature
- 1½ tablespoons fresh lemon juice (about ½ lemon)
- 1½ teaspoons lemon zest (about ½ lemon)
- 1 teaspoon vanilla extract
- 1/3 cup powdered monk fruit sweetener (or powdered / confectioners' sweetener of choice)
- 1 cup almond flour, + 2 tablespoons (measured correctly with the spoon and level method)
- For the Glaze:
- 1/3 cup powdered monk fruit sweetener (or powdered / confectioners' sweetener of choice)
- 2-3 teaspoons almond milk or milk of your choice

Directions

1. Preheat the oven to 350°F. Line a baking sheet with parchment paper and set aside.
2. In the bowl of an electric mixer fitted with a paddle attachment, beat the butter on high until light and creamy.
3. Add the lemon juice and lemon zest and mix until combined.
4. On low speed, gradually add blanched almond flour then powdered monk fruit sweetener and vanilla and mix until the dough comes together.
5. Use a medium cookie scoop (or manually measure 1.5 tablespoon balls), scoop out 9 cookies, and transfer to the prepared sheet. If the dough seems too wet, add up to 1 tablespoon of almond flour.

6. Bake approximately 8-10 minutes or until just browned around bottom edges.
7. Transfer to wire racks; let cool completely.
8. While the cookies are cooling, make the glaze. In a medium bowl, whisk together powdered sweetener and milk. Drizzle over cooled cookies and enjoy immediately or place in the refrigerator until set.

Nutrition: Per serving (1 cookie) | Calories: 132 | Total Fats: 12g | Carbohydrates: 2g | Fiber: 1g | Protein: 2g

51. Peanut Butter Cups

Preparation Time: 10 minutes + 20-25 minutes Chill Time
Cooking Time: 1 minute
Serving: 16 cups

Ingredients:
- 1 cup sugar-free chocolate chips, like Lily's
- 1 tablespoon coconut oil
- ½ cup peanut butter
- 2 tablespoons powdered erythritol sweetener, optional
- ¼ teaspoon salt, optional

Directions:
1. Line a muffin tin with 16 silicone liners. Set aside.
2. Melt the chocolate chips and coconut oil together in the microwave on 50% power in 20-second increments until completely melted, stirring after each burst. You can also melt the chocolate chips with oil over a double boiler, if you prefer.
3. Measure 1 teaspoon of the melted chocolate into each silicone cup, reserving the remaining chocolate. Swirl the chocolate up around the sides of the cups to coat them.
4. Place in the freezer for 10 minutes so the chocolate can set.
5. Put the peanut butter in a heat safe bowl and microwave in quick bursts of 15 seconds until the peanut butter is liquid and pourable. (If your peanut butter is already liquid at room temperature, you can skip this step.)
6. Add optional sweetener and optional salt to the peanut butter and stir to combine.
7. Remove muffin tin from freezer.
8. Spoon about 1 teaspoon of melted peanut butter over chocolate in each cup. Tap the cups on the counter to smooth the tops of the peanut butter cups.

9. Spoon the rest of the chocolate over the top of the peanut butter, making sure the peanut butter layer is completely covered.

10. Return muffin tin to freezer for 10-15 minutes.

11. Store refrigerated in an airtight container for 3 days.

Nutrition: Per serving (1 cup) | Calories: 60 | Total Fats: 5g | Carbohydrates: 2g | Fiber: 1g | Protein: 2g | Sugar: 1g

52. Lemon Mug Cake

Preparation Time: 5 minutes

Cooking Time: about 2 minutes

Serving: 1

Ingredients

- 1 egg regular size
- 4 tablespoons almond flour
- ½ teaspoon baking powder
- 1½ tablespoons erythritol or Monk Fruit or Xylitol
- 2 tablespoons lemon juice
- 1 teaspoon grated lemon zest
- 2 tablespoons blueberries-fresh or frozen (optional)*

Directions

1. Break the egg into a small mixing bowl, add the almond flour, baking powder, sugar free crystal sweetener and lemon juice, and whisk until a consistent cake batter is formed.
2. Add lemon zest and blueberries, if desired.
3. Pour the batter into a tall microwave safe mug. Your mug cake is going to rise and double in height, so make sure the mug you use is tall enough to keep the mug cake batter from overflowing in the microwave. Don't microwave into 2 mugs, or it will impact the microwaving time consequently. Bake all at once and share!
4. Cook in microwave on high (800 w) for about 90 seconds.
5. Allow to cool for 2-3 minutes and then eat directly out of mug or remove carefully to a plate.

*****Note:** Nutrition info does not include optional blueberries.

Nutrition: Per serving (1 mug cake) I Calories: 240 I Total Fats: 9.9g I Carbohydrates: 8.6g I Fiber: 1.2g I Protein: 10.4g I Sugar: 1g

53. Mint Ice Cream

Preparation Time: 15 minutes

Chilling Time: 2 hours

Cooking Time: 0 minutes

Serving: 2

Ingredients

- ½ cup full-fat coconut milk
- ½ medium avocado
- ½ teaspoon vanilla extract
- ½-¾ teaspoon peppermint extract or to taste
- ½ teaspoon lemon juice, freshly squeezed
- Pinch flakey sea salt or salt of choice
- 3 tablespoons powdered xylitol or sweetener of choice or to taste
- 1-1.5 ounces sugar-free chocolate chips (optional)*

Directions

1. If your coconut milk has the solids and liquids separated, pop it in a quick water bath until everything comes together. Be sure it's back at room temp before blending.
2. Place coconut milk, avocado, vanilla extract, peppermint extract, lemon juice, salt and sweetener in a blender and blend on high until completely creamy and smooth.
3. Fold in the chocolate chips (see note) then transfer ice cream to a sealable container, cover the surface with plastic wrap, and freeze until set, about 2 hours.
4. To serve, simply remove from the freezer for 15 minutes or so to soften it enough to make it "scoopable".
5. Enjoy!

*Note: Nutritional Facts do not include optional chocolate chips.

Nutrition: Per serving (1 scoop) | Calories: 151 | Total Fats: 15g | Carbohydrates: 3.5g | Fiber: 2g | Protein: 1.5g

CONCLUSION

This cookbook is intended for use by vegetarians who want to enjoy their vegetarian lifestyle without feeling deprived or starving. It's also ideal for those who must adhere to a vegetarian diet but still wish to eat well and/or lose weight.

The recipes in this book are largely vegan, meaning they don't contain eggs, dairy, or honey. They do not include meat or fish for the most part either (we make some exceptions).

In a nutshell, the goal of this cookbook is to provide vegetarians with nutritious, uncomplicated meals that they can enjoy.

This book is a great resource for people who want to improve their health by adopting a vegetarian lifestyle but still want to enjoy their favorite foods – like pizza, desserts, etc.... without giving in to temptations. This book's recipes were picked with care since they are: Easy to follow and quick to make – no need for special ingredients or cooking techniques, nor expensive/complicated kitchenware. Many of these dishes are so simple to make that even children can do it (they will surely find it fun too).

High in nutrition, so you will feel full and satisfied after eating your meals. These recipes are nutrient-dense, and contain healthy fats that assist weight loss.

Easy to prepare at home – no need to spend hours preparing special meals on special days, or having a car trip to the nearest restaurant which may not be vegan (for some cuisines it just won't work). This cookbook is ideal for those who have never cooked or baked before.

Quick and easy to prepare at home – especially when you are on a short time schedule. Even youngsters can create the dishes because they are so simple to make, especially if they are permitted to try the dish beforehand.

Healthy – the recipes are healthy and nutritious, avoiding certain ingredients that aren't good for health, such as refined sugar and unhealthy fats.

Delicious – most of the recipe in this book have been chosen because they taste great, and people enjoy them intensely.

The recipes in this cookbook can suit people at all stages of life, from kids to seniors. It's critical not to overlook meals and snacks that are appropriate for special diets, especially if you or a member of your family follows one.

The 30-Minute
Vegetarian Keto Cookbook

Delicious Keto Friendly Vegetarian Recipes that You Can Cook Under 30-Minute

ANNA PRENTICE

INTRODUCTION

If you're a vegetarian, or trying to be one, the ketogenic diet is likely something you've researched. However, sometimes it's hard to find good recipes that are both vegan and low-carb. On this site, you'll find over 100 vegan keto recipes covering breakfast, lunch/dinner and snacks for every day of the week.

Yes! There is no excuse not to try out a new veggie-based meal with these recipes and learn how meatless dinners can actually taste amazing! We searched high and low for any recipe that was not already uploaded in our archive; we also include cooking tips for those who may be new to the ketogenic lifestyle.

Here's my personal advice for anyone who is trying the ketogenic diet. Do not think that you need meat to do the keto diet, in fact, completely removing meat from your meals frees up a lot of calories, making it easier to be more in control of what ingredients you use. Also, if you are used to eating meals with a lot of carbohydrates, it will take time to re-program your brain to get used of eating fats and proteins instead; this will take a few days of getting used to. Don't give up though! Once you get used to eating foods with more fat and protein, you will be able to feel fuller longer, so your hunger will decrease. Try it! Ketogenic diet is simply amazing.

Humans can have a low carb diet by eating in a way that is much healthier for the body than conventional diets. Whether it be from Keto recipes or vegan recipes, these simple foods can have a huge difference on your status in the body. By switching over to a low carb and fat-based diet you will be able to take advantage of many other benefits as well such as weight loss or simply just feeling better overall.

As you search for low carb vegan keto recipes you must look for ingredients that are high in fats. This will make following a vegetarian or vegan ketogenic diet much easier. If you have allergies or your own reasons for not eating something that is certain to have lots of carbs then this may be very difficult for you. When following these kinds of diets, it's essential to prioritize your health.

Vegetarian and Vegan recipes can be made in a way that can help anyone on the Low Carb High Fat diet feel great about their food choices as they lose weight or just eat healthier. It is important that you get many different kinds of vegetables into your diet to help with your overall health and wellbeing. This is why adding in recipes like these can be so beneficial, as they will make it simple for you to prepare delicious meals.

When you need a recipe one of the best options that you have is to make one yourself. This can be a great way for you to make something that fits your own wants and needs perfectly. It can also save money if you are looking to keep costs down. This can be great for you as you get used to eating this new style of food.

RECIPES FOR BREAKFAST

1. Almond Cinnamon Smoothie

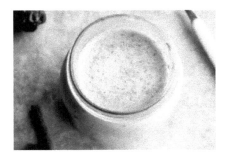

Preparation Time: 10 minutes

Cooking Time: 15 minutes

Servings: 1

Ingredients:

- ¾ cup almond milk, unsweetened
- ¼ cup coconut oil
- 1 tablespoon almond butter, unsweetened
- 1 tablespoon vanilla protein powder
- 1/8 teaspoon cinnamon

Directions:

1. Add into your blender all the ingredients, blend them until they are nice and smooth. Serve and enjoy!

Nutritional Values (Per Serving): Calories: 500 Fat: 43 g Carbohydrates: 10 g Sugar: 2 g Protein: 14.6 g Cholesterol: 0 mg

2. Almond Flour Waffles

Preparation Time: 10 minutes

Cooking Time: 5 minutes

Servings: 2

Ingredients:

- Pinch of xanthan gum
- Pinch of salt
- 1 tablespoon butter, melted
- 1 large organic egg
- 2 tablespoons sour cream
- 1 teaspoon vinegar
- 2 teaspoons arrowroot flour
- 1/8 teaspoon baking powder
- 1/8 teaspoon baking soda
- ¼ cup almond flour

Directions:

1. In a mixing bowl combine vinegar, butter, sour cream, and egg mix well. Add dry ingredients into wet and mix until well blended. Heat your waffle iron and cook waffle for 5 minutes or to your waffle iron instructions. Serve and enjoy!

Nutritional Values (Per Serving): Calories: 208 Fat: 18 g Carbohydrates: 4.83 g Sugar: 2.1 g Protein: 6.52 g Cholesterol: 114 mg

3. <u>Healthy Breakfast Porridge</u>

Preparation Time: 5 minutes

Cooking Time: 5 minutes

Servings: 2

Ingredients:

- 1/8 teaspoon salt
- 4 tablespoons coconut, unsweetened, shredded
- 1 tablespoon oat bran
- 1 tablespoon flaxseed meal
- ½ tablespoon butter
- ¾ teaspoon Truvia
- ½ teaspoon cinnamon
- ½ cup heavy cream
- 1 cup water

Directions:

1. Add all your ingredients into a saucepan over medium-low heat. Once the mixture comes to a boil remove from heat. Serve warm and enjoy!

Nutritional Values (Per Serving): Calories: 222 Fat: 21 g Carbohydrates: 3.90 g Sugar: 3.9 g Protein: 2.68 g, Cholesterol: 49 mg

4. Parsley Spread

Preparation time: 5 minutes

Cooking time: 0 minutes

Servings: 8

Ingredients:

- 1 cup parsley leaves
- 1 cup coconut cream
- 1 tablespoon sun-dried tomatoes, chopped
- 2 tablespoons lime juice
- ¼ cup shallots, chopped
- 1 teaspoon oregano, dried
- A pinch of salt and black pepper

Directions:

1. In a blender, combine the parsley with the cream, the tomatoes and the other ingredients, pulse well, divide into bowls and serve for breakfast.

Nutrition: calories 78, fat 7.2, fiber 1, carbs 3.6, protein 1.1

5. Baked Cheesy Artichokes

Preparation time: 10 minutes

Cooking time: 45 minutes

Servings: 6

Ingredients:

- 1 cup spinach, chopped
- 1 cup almond milk
- 12 ounces canned artichokes, halved
- 2 garlic cloves, minced
- ½ cup cashew cheese, shredded
- 1 tablespoon dill, chopped
- A pinch of salt and black pepper
- teaspoons olive oil

Directions:

1. Heat up a pan with the oil over medium heat, add the garlic, artichokes, salt and pepper, stir and cook for 5 minutes.

2. Transfer this to a baking dish, add the spinach, almond milk and the other ingredients, toss a bit, bake at 380 degrees F for 40 minutes, divide between plates and serve for breakfast.

Nutrition: calories 149, fat 12.2, fiber 4.3, carbs 9.7, protein 3.5

6. Cauliflower Couscous

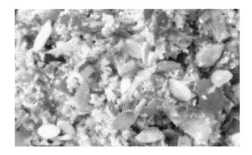

Preparation Time: 10 minutes

Cooking Time: 10 minutes

Servings: 3

Ingredients

- ½ head cauliflower, pulsed in food processor
- 3-4 kale leaves, de-stemmed, chopped
- oz. sun dried tomatoes, drained
- ¼ cup olives - 1 garlic clove, crushed
- 3 Tbsp. olive oil - 1 Tbsp. lemon juice
- ½ tsp cumin, ground - 1 tsp oregano, dried
- Salt and pepper to taste
- Tofu, crumbled for topping (about 1 Tbsp. per plate)
- Basil, chopped for topping (about 1 Tbsp. per plate)

Directions

1. In a preheated pan with olive oil, add garlic and kale. Cook for 2 minutes, stirring.

2. Add cauliflower and season with salt.

3. Add the remaining ingredients and spices and cook for 2-3 minutes, stirring.

4. Top with tofu and basil.

Nutrition: Carbs: 8 g Fat: 11 g Protein: 4 g Calories: 145

7. Fried Eggplant

Preparation Time: 5 minutes

Cooking Time: 25 minutes

Servings: 4

Ingredients

- 2 eggplants, rinsed, cut in circles
- 3-4 garlic cloves, crushed
- Salt and pepper to taste
- ½ cup vegetable oil

Directions

1. Season eggplant circles with salt and pepper.
2. In a preheated pan with 2 Tbsp. oil, add eggplant circles in one layer.
3. Fry for 1-2 minutes on each side until golden.
4. Transfer to a plate and sprinkle with crushed garlic.
5. Repeat with the remaining eggplants, adding more oil to a pan between batches.

Nutrition: Carbs: 16 g Fat: 25.7 g Protein: 3 g Calories: 294

8. Eggplant & Tomatoes Salad

Preparation Time: 25 minutes

Cooking Time: 10 minutes

Servings: 4

Ingredients

- 2 eggplants, cut in circles
- 2 red bell peppers, deseeded, cut in rings
- 3 tomatoes, cut in semi circles
- 1 onion, cut in semi circles
- 5-10 sprigs fresh parsley, chopped
- Salt and pepper to taste
- Olive oil (for frying the eggplants + salad dressing)

Directions

1. Season eggplant circles with salt and let stand in a bowl while preparing the other ingredients.
2. After all other vegetables are chopped, drain the eggplants and place in a preheated pan with oil. Fry on both sides until golden, 1-2 minutes per side.
3. Combine the vegetables in a salad bowl, add chopped parsley, and dress with oil. Serve.

Nutrition: Carbs: 16 g Fat: 11.3 g Protein: 4.9 g Calories: 113

9. Eggplant Pate

Preparation Time: 15 minutes

Cooking Time: 1 hour

Servings: 4

Ingredients

- 3-4 eggplants, peeled, cubed - 4 bell peppers, cubed
- 3 tomatoes, cubed - 2 onions, cubed
- 2-3 garlic cloves, minced - A bunch of parsley, chopped
- 3 Tbsp. olive oil - Salt and pepper to taste

Directions

1. Season eggplants with salt and let stand in a bowl while preparing other vegetables.
2. Combine all ingredients in a Crockpot. Season with salt and pepper. Add oil and stir.
3. Select the "Stew" mode and cook for 1 hour, covered.
4. After an hour, puree the cooked vegetables with a blender. Remove the excess liquid if there is any.

Nutrition: Carbs: 15 g Fat: 10.8 g Protein: 2.5 g Calories: 165

10. Pickled Eggplant

Preparation Time: 24 hours

Cooking Time: 25 minutes

Servings: 4

Ingredients

- 2 eggplants, peeled, sliced - 1 large onion
- 2-3 garlic cloves, crushed - 1 tsp salt
- 1 tsp Keto friendly sweetener
- 2 Tbsp. vegetable oil + more for baking
- 1 Tbsp. vinegar
- 3 sprigs parsley, chopped

Directions

1. Arrange the eggplants on a baking dish in one layer and oil them.
2. Bake in the oven at 350F for 25 minutes.
3. In a bowl, combine onions, garlic, parsley, salt, sweetener, oil, and vinegar.
4. Chop the baked eggplant and drop into the brine.
5. Transfer to a jar, cover with lid, and refrigerate for 24 hours.

Nutrition: Carbs: 18 g Fat: 7 g Protein: 3.6 g Calories: 158

RECIPES FOR DINNER

11. Tamarind Avocado Bowls

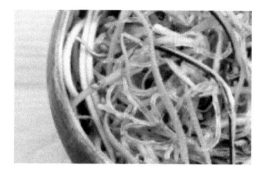

Preparation Time: 10 minutes

Cooking Time: 0 minutes

Servings: 2

Ingredients:

- 1 teaspoon cumin seeds

- 1 tablespoon olive oil

- ½ teaspoon gram masala

- 1 teaspoon ground ginger

- 2 avocados, peeled, pitted and roughly cubed

- 1 mango, peeled, and cubed

- 1 cup cherry tomatoes, halved

- ½ teaspoon cayenne pepper

- 1 teaspoon turmeric powder

- 3 tablespoons tamarind paste

Directions:

1. In a bowl, mix the avocados with the mango and the other ingredients, toss and serve.

Nutrition: Calories 170 Fat 4.5 Fiber 3 Carbs 5 Protein 6

12. Avocado and Leeks Mix

Preparation Time: 10 minutes

Cooking Time: 0 minutes

Servings: 4

Ingredients:

- 1 small red onion, chopped
- 2 avocados, pitted, peeled and chopped
- 1 teaspoon chili powder
- 2 leeks, sliced
- 1 cup cucumber, cubed
- 1 cup cherry tomatoes, halved
- Salt and black pepper to the taste
- 2 tablespoons cumin powder
- 2 tablespoons lime juice
- 1 tablespoon parsley, chopped

Directions:

1. In a bowl, mix the onion with the avocados, chili powder and the other ingredients, toss and serve.

Nutrition: Calories 120 Fat 2 Fiber 2 Carbs 7 Protein 4

13. Cabbage Bowls

Preparation Time: 10 minutes

Cooking Time: 10 minutes

Servings: 4

Ingredients:

- 1 green cabbage head, shredded
- 1 red cabbage head, shredded
- 1 teaspoon garam masala
- 1 teaspoon basil, dried
- 1 teaspoon coriander, ground
- 1 teaspoon mustard seeds
- 1 tablespoon balsamic vinegar
- ¼ cup tomatoes, crushed
- A pinch of salt and black pepper
- 3 carrots, shredded
- 1 yellow bell pepper, chopped
- 1 orange bell pepper, chopped
- 1 red bell pepper, chopped
- 2 tablespoons dill, chopped
- 2 tablespoons olive oil

Directions:

1. Heat up a pan with the oil over medium heat, add the peppers and carrots and cook for 2 minutes.
2. Add the cabbage and the other ingredients, toss, cook for 10 minutes, divide between plates and serve.

Nutrition: Calories 150 Fat 9 Fiber 4 Carbs 3.3 Protein 4.4

14. Pomegranate and Pears Salad

Preparation Time: 10 minutes

Cooking Time: 0 minutes

Servings: 3

Ingredients:

- 3 big pears, cored and cut with a spiralizer
- ¾ cup pomegranate seeds
- 2 cups baby spinach
- ½ cup black olives, pitted and cubed
- ¾ cup walnuts, chopped1 tablespoon olive oil
- 1 tablespoon coconut sugar
- 1 teaspoon white sesame seeds
- 2 tablespoons chives, chopped
- 1 tablespoon balsamic vinegar
- 1 garlic clove, minced
- A pinch of sea salt and black pepper

Directions:

1. In a bowl, mix the pears with the pomegranate seeds, spinach and the other ingredients, toss and serve.

Nutrition: Calories 200 Fat 3.9 Fiber 4 Carbs 6 Protein 3.3

15. Bulgur and Tomato Mix

Preparation Time: 15 minutes

Cooking Time: 0 minutes

Servings: 4

Ingredients:

- 1 ½ cups hot water
- 1 cup bulgur
- Juice of 1 lime
- 1 cup cherry tomatoes, halved
- 4 tablespoons cilantro, chopped
- ½ cup cranberries, dried
- juice of ½ lemon
- 1 teaspoon oregano, dried
- 1/3 cup almonds, sliced
- ¼ cup green onions, chopped
- ½ cup red bell peppers, chopped
- ½ cup carrots, grated
- 1 tablespoon avocado oil
- A pinch of sea salt and black pepper

Directions:

1. Place bulgur into a bowl, add boiling water to it, stir, and cover and set aside for 15 minutes.

2. Fluff bulgur with a fork and transfer to a bowl.

3. Add the rest of the ingredients, toss and serve.

Nutrition: Calories 260 Fat 4.4 Fiber 3 Carbs 7 Protein 10

RECIPES FOR VEGAN AND VEGETABLES

16. Wok Fried Broccoli

Preparation Time: 10 minutes

Cooking Time: 16 minutes

Servings: 02

Ingredients:

- 3 ounces whole, blanched peanuts
- 2 tablespoons olive oil
- 1 banana shallot, sliced
- 10 ounces broccoli, trimmed and cut into florets
- ¼ red pepper, julienned
- ½ yellow pepper, julienned
- 1 teaspoon soy sauce

Directions:

1. Toast peanuts on a baking sheet for 15 minutes at 350 degrees F.
2. In a wok, add oil and shallots and sauté for 10 minutes.
3. Toss in broccoli and peppers.
4. Stir fry for 3 minutes then add the rest of the ingredients.
5. Cook for 3 additional minutes and serve.

Nutrition: Calories: 391 Total Fat: 39g Carbs: 15g Net Carbs: 5g Fiber: 2g Protein: 6g

17. Broccoli & Brown Rice Satay

Preparation Time: 10 minutes

Cooking Time: 10 minutes

Servings: 4

Ingredients:

- 6 trimmed broccoli florets, halved
- 1-inch piece of ginger, shredded
- 2 garlic cloves, shredded
- 1 red onion, sliced
- 1 roasted red pepper, cut into cubes
- 2 teaspoons olive oil
- 1 teaspoon mild chili powder
- 1 tablespoon reduced salt soy sauce
- 1 tablespoon maple syrup
- 1 cup cooked brown rice

Directions:

1. Boil broccoli in water for 4 minutes then drain immediately.
2. In a pan add olive oil, ginger, onion, and garlic.
3. Stir fry for 2 minutes then add the rest of the ingredients.
4. Cook for 3 minutes then serve.

Nutrition: Calories: 196 Total Fat: 20g Carbs: 8g Net Carbs: 3g Fiber: 1g Protein: 3g

18. Sautéed Sesame Spinach

Preparation Time: 1 hr. 10 minutes

Cooking Time: 3 minutes

Servings: 04

Ingredients:

- 1 tablespoon toasted sesame oil
- ½ tablespoon soy sauce
- ½ teaspoon toasted sesame seeds, crushed
- ½ teaspoon rice vinegar
- ½ teaspoon golden caster sugar
- 1 garlic clove, grated
- 8 ounces spinach, stem ends trimmed

Directions:

1. Sauté spinach in a pan until it is wilted.
2. Whisk the sesame oil, garlic, sugar, vinegar, sesame seeds, soy sauce and black pepper together in a bowl.
3. Stir in spinach and mix well.
4. Cover and refrigerate for 1 hour.
5. Serve.

Nutrition: Calories: 677 Total Fat: 60g Carbs: 71g Net Carbs: 7g Fiber: 0g; Protein: 20g

19. Mimosa Salad

Preparation Time: 10 Minutes

Cooking Time: 0 Minutes

Servings: 8

Ingredients:

- Mint, fresh, one half cup

- Orange juice, one half cup

- Pineapple, one cup cut into small pieces

- Strawberries, one cup cut into quarters

- Blueberries, one cup

- Blackberries, one cup

- Kiwi, three peeled and sliced

Directions:

1. In a large-sized bowl, mix all of the fruits together and then top with the orange juice and the fresh mint.

2. Toss gently together all of the fruit until they are well mixed.

Nutrition: Calories: 215 Protein: 3g Fat: 1g Carbs: 49g

20. Honey Lime Quinoa Fruit Salad

Preparation Time: 20 Minutes

Cooking Time: 0 Minutes

Servings: 6

Ingredients:

- Basil, chopped, one tablespoon
- Lime juice, two tablespoons
- Mango, diced, one cup
- Blueberries, one cup
- Blackberries, one cup
- Strawberries, sliced, one- and one-half cup
- Quinoa, cooked, one cup

Directions:

1. In a large-sized bowl, mix the fruits with the cooked quinoa and mix well.

2. Drizzle on the lime juice and add the chopped basil and mix the fruit gently but thoroughly to coat all of the pieces.

Nutrition: Calories: 246 Protein: 7g Fat: 1g Carbs: 44g

SIDES DISH

21. Carrot and Soy Bean Stir Fry

Preparation Time: 15 minutes

Cooking Time: 20 minutes

Servings: 2

Ingredients:

- ¼ cup cauliflower florets
- ¼ cup broccoli florets
- 1/2 cup dried soybeans
- 1 large carrot, chopped
- ½ cup vegetable broth
- 1 tablespoon butter
- 1 onion, chopped
- ½ cup pumpkin, sliced
- 2 large mushrooms, sliced
- 1 tablespoon garlic powder
- Salt and pepper to taste

Directions:

1. Select the Sauté setting on the Instant Pot, add the butter, and heat for 1 minute. Add the onions, carrots, garlic powder, salt, pumpkin, broccoli, cauliflower, and

mushrooms. Sauté for about 10 minutes, until the vegetables give up some of their liquid and begin to brown just a bit.

2. Add vegetable broth and soybeans.

3. Lock the lid into place. Select Pressure Cook or Manual, and adjust the pressure to High and the time to 12 minutes. After cooking, let the pressure release naturally for 10 minutes, then quickly release any remaining pressure.

4. Unlock the lid.

5. Taste the soybeans and adjust the seasoning.

6. Serve and enjoy.

Nutrition: Calories 291, Total Fat 5. 2g, Saturated Fat 3.1g, Cholesterol 0mg, Sodium 1089mg, Total Carbohydrate 13.7g, Dietary Fiber 4. 6g, Total Sugars 1g, Protein 22. 4g

22. Tomato Chickpeas Curry

Preparation Time: 15 minutes

Cooking Time: 20 minutes

Servings: 2

Ingredients:

- 1 tablespoon avocado oil
- 5 tomatoes, cored and diced
- 1 1/2 teaspoons garlic powder
- ½ tablespoon coarsely chopped fresh rosemary
- 1½ cups chickpeas drained and rinsed
- ½ teaspoon kosher salt
- Freshly ground black pepper
- 3 cups of water

Directions:

1. Select the Sauté setting on the Instant Pot, add the avocado oil. Add the tomatoes and sauté for about 3 minutes until they start to break down and tomatoes become saucy. Add the garlic powder, rosemary and sauté for 1 minute more.

2. Add water and chickpeas, salt, and pepper.

3. Lock the lid into place. Select Pressure Cook or Manual, and adjust the pressure to High and the time to 12

minutes. After cooking, let the pressure release naturally for 10 minutes, then quickly release any remaining pressure.

4. Unlock the lid.

5. Serve and enjoy.

Nutrition: Calories 434, Total Fat 7.6g, Saturated Fat 0.9g, Cholesterol 0mg, Sodium 621mg, Total Carbohydrate 74 1g, Dietary Fiber 21. 6g, Total Sugars 19.2g, Protein 22. 4g

23. Lemony Lentil and Greens

Preparation Time: 10 minutes

Cooking Time: 25 minutes

Servings: 2

Ingredients:

- ½ cup brown lentils, rinsed
- ½ tablespoon butter
- 1 onion, diced
- ½ cup kale, chopped
- 2 cups vegetable broth
- Juice of 1 lemon
- 1/4 teaspoon paprika

Directions:

1. Select the Sauté setting on the Instant Pot, add the butter, onions, sprinkle with a pinch of sea salt, and cook for 1 minute.

2. Next, add the chopped kale and paprika then stir together. Cook for another 2 minutes until the kale is slightly soft. Add the brown lentils to the Instant Pot along with the vegetable broth.

3. Lock the lid into place. Select Pressure Cook or Manual, and adjust the pressure to High and the time

to 20 minutes. After cooking, let the pressure release naturally for 10 minutes, then quickly release any remaining pressure. Unlock the lid.

4.   Squeeze the juice of a lemon into the pot and stir together.

Nutrition: Calories 264, Total Fat 4. 9g, Saturated Fat 2.3g, Cholesterol 8mg, Sodium 798mg, Total Carbohydrate 36.8g, Dietary Fiber 16.2g, Total Sugars 4g, Protein 18. 4g

24. Moroccan Red Lentil Curry

Preparation Time: 10 minutes

Cooking Time: 30 minutes

Servings: 2

Ingredients:

- ½ cup dry red lentils
- ½ leek, diced
- 1 small onion, diced
- ½ zucchini, peeled and chopped
- 1 potato, peeled and chopped
- ½ teaspoon garlic powder
- 1 tablespoon coconut oil
- ½ teaspoon cumin
- ½ teaspoon turmeric powder
- ¼ teaspoon coriander powder
- ¼ teaspoon nutmeg
- 2 cups vegetable broth
- Juice of ½ lemon
- Salt to taste (if needed
- Fresh cilantro for topping

Directions:

1. Select Sauté and adjust to Normal or Medium heat. Add the coconut oil to the Instant Pot and heat until shimmering. Add onions and the leeks. Cook for 2 minutes.

2. Next add the zucchini, garlic powder, and potatoes along with the spices. Stir together and cook for 1 minute then pour in vegetable broth.

3. Add red lentils. Lock the lid into place. Select Pressure Cook or Manual, and adjust the pressure to High and the time to 20 minutes. After cooking, let the pressure release naturally for 10 minutes, then quickly release any remaining pressure.

4. Unlock the lid. Squeeze in the lemon juice and stir together. Garnish with fresh cilantro.

Nutrition: Calories 383, Total Fat 9. 3g, Saturated Fat 6.5g, Cholesterol 0mg, Sodium 784mg, Total Carbohydrate 56.6g, Dietary Fiber 19 3g, Total Sugars 6 5g, Protein 20. 9g

25. White Bean Spinach & Tomato Curry

Preparation Time: 15 minutes

Cooking Time: 25 minutes

Servings: 2

Ingredients:

- 1 teaspoon vegetable oil
- 1 small onion, diced
- 1 zucchini, peeled and diced
- ½ teaspoon garlic, powder
- ½ teaspoon dried basil
- ¼ teaspoon salt
- ¼ teaspoon pepper
- 1/2 teaspoon crushed red pepper
- ½ cup spinach chopped
- 1 cup white beans, drained and rinsed
- ½ cup tomatoes
- 1 1/2 cups vegetable broth

Directions:

1. Select the Sauté setting on the Instant Pot, add the vegetable oil, and heat for 1 minute. Add the onion and sauté for 2 minutes, then add the zucchini, garlic

powder, tomatoes, and seasonings (salt, pepper, and basil) and continue to sauté for another 2 minutes.

2. Add the spinach to the Instant Pot and cook until it starts to wilt. Pour vegetable broth and white beans.

3. Select Pressure Cook or Manual, and adjust the pressure to High and the time to 20 minutes. After cooking, let the pressure release naturally for 10 minutes, then quickly release any remaining pressure.

4. Unlock the lid and serve.

Nutrition: Calories 418, Total Fat 4. 2g, Saturated Fat 0 9g, Cholesterol 0mg, Sodium 708mg, Total Carbohydrate 70 6g, Dietary Fiber 18 1g, Total Sugars 6 9g, Protein 28. 3g

RECIPES FOR PASTA

26. Fresh Tomato Mint Pasta

Preparation Time:05 minutes

Cooking Time: 10 minutes

Servings: 2

Ingredients:

- 1 cup pasta
- 1 tablespoon coconut oil
- ½ teaspoon garlic powder
- 1 tomato
- ½ tablespoon butter
- ¼ cup fresh mint
- ¼ cup of coconut milk
- Salt & pepper to taste
- Enough water

Directions:

1. Add the coconut oil to the Instant Pot hit "Sauté", add in the garlic, and stir. Add the tomatoes and a pinch of salt. Then add mint and pepper.

2. Next, add coconut milk, butter, and water. Stir well, lastly, add in the pasta.

3. Secure the lid and hit "Keep Warm/Cancel" and then hit "Manual" or "Pressure Cook" High Pressure for 6 minutes. Quick-release when done.

4. Enjoy.

Nutrition: Calories 350, Total Fat 18. 5g, Saturated Fat 14 3g, Cholesterol 54mg, Sodium 47mg, Total Carbohydrate 39 4g, Dietary Fiber 1.9g, Total Sugars 2g, Protein 8. 7g

27. Corn and Chiles Fusilli

Preparation Time:05 minutes

Cooking Time: 05 minutes

Servings: 2

Ingredients:

- ½ tablespoon butter
- 1 tablespoon garlic minced
- Salt and pepper to taste
- 2 oz. can green chills
- ½ cup frozen corn kernels
- ¼ teaspoon cumin
- 1/8 teaspoon paprika
- 1 cup fusilli
- 1 cup vegetable broth
- ¼ cup coconut cream
- 2 leeks, sliced
- 1/8 bunch parsley
- 1 oz. shredded mozzarella cheese

Directions:

1. In the Instant Pot, add butter when butter melt, place the minced garlic, salt, and pepper, then press Sauté on the

Instant Pot. Add the can of green chills (with juices), frozen corn kernels, cumin, and paprika.

2. Add the uncooked fusilli and vegetable broth to the Instant Pot.

3. Place the lid on the Instant Pot, and bring the toggle switch into the "Sealing" position. Press Manual or Pressure Cook and adjust the time for 5 minutes.

4. When the five minutes are up, do a Natural-release for 5 minutes and then move the toggle switch to "Venting" to release the rest of the pressure in the pot.

5. Remove the lid. If the mixture looks watery, press "Sauté", and bring the mixture up to a boil and let it boil for a few minutes. Then add the coconut cream and stir until it has fully coated the pasta. Stir in most of the sliced leek and parsley, reserving a little to sprinkle over top, mozzarella on top of the pasta.

Nutrition: Calories 399, Total Fat 14. 4g, Saturated Fat 10g, Cholesterol 15mg, Sodium 531mg, Total Carbohydrate 56.2g, Dietary Fiber 4.9g, Total Sugars 7 2g, Protein 15. 4g

28. Creamy Penne with Vegetables

Preparation Time:05 minutes

Cooking Time: 10 minutes

Servings: 2

Ingredients:

- ½ tablespoon butter
- 1 cup penne
- 1 small onion
- ½ teaspoon garlic powder
- 1 carrot
- ½ red bell pepper
- ½ pumpkin
- 2 cups vegetable broth
- 2 oz. coconut cream
- 1/8 cup grated Parmesan cheese
- 1/8 teaspoon salt and pepper to taste
- Dash hot sauce, optional
- ¼ cup cauliflower florets

Directions:

1. Set Instant Pot to Sauté. Add the butter and allow it to melt. Add the onion and garlic powder and cook for 2

minutes. Stir regularly. Add the carrot, red pepper and pumpkin, and cauliflower to the pot.

2. Add penne, vegetable broth, coconut cream, salt, and pepper then add hot sauce.

3. Lock the lid and make sure the vent is closed. Set Instant Pot to Manual or Pressure Cook on High Pressure for 10 minutes. When cooking time ends, release pressure and wait for steam to completely stop before opening the lid.

4. Stir in cheese, sprinkle a bit on top of the pasta when you serve it.

Nutrition: Calories 381, Total Fat 13. 2g, Saturated Fat 8.7g, Cholesterol 56mg, Sodium 1006mg, Total Carbohydrate 52 3g, Dietary Fiber 4 7g, Total Sugars 8.6g, Protein 15. 3g

29. Pasta with Eggplant Sauce

Preparation Time:05 minutes

Cooking Time: 10 minutes

Servings: 2

Ingredients:

- 1 tablespoon coconut oil
- 2 cloves garlic
- 1 small onion
- 1 medium eggplant
- 1 cup diced tomatoes
- 1 tablespoon tomato sauce
- ¼ teaspoon dried thyme
- ½ teaspoon honey
- Pinch paprika
- Freshly cracked pepper
- ¼ salt and pepper, or to taste
- 6 oz. spaghetti
- 2 cups vegetable broth
- Handful fresh coriander, chopped

Directions:

1. Set Instant Pot to Sauté. Add the coconut oil and allow it to melt. Add the onion and garlic and cook for 2 minutes or until the onion is soft and transparent.

2. Add eggplant, diced tomatoes, tomato sauce, thyme, honey, paprika, and freshly cracked pepper. Stir them well to combine, Add spaghetti, and vegetable broth, salt, and pepper.

3. Lock the lid and make sure the vent is closed. Set Instant Pot to Manual or Pressure Cook on High Pressure for 10 minutes. When cooking time ends, release pressure and wait for steam to completely stop before opening the lid.

4. Top each serving with grated goat and a sprinkle of fresh coriander.

Nutrition: Calories 306, Total Fat 18g, Saturated Fat 12. 9g, Cholesterol 30mg, Sodium 188mg, Total Carbohydrate 27g, Dietary Fiber 12.6g 45%, Total Sugars 13 9g, Protein 14.2g

30. Creamy Pesto Pasta with Tofu & Broccoli

Preparation Time:05 minutes

Cooking Time: 10 minutes

Servings: 2

Ingredients:

- 4 oz. Farfalle pasta
- 4 oz. frozen broccoli florets
- ½ tablespoon coconut oil
- ½ cup tofu
- ¼ cup basil pesto
- ¼ cup vegetable broth
- 2 oz. heavy cream

Directions:

1. In the Instant Pot, add Farfalline pasta, broccoli, coconut oil, tofu, basil pesto, vegetable broth. Cover the Instant Pot and lock it in.

2. Set the Manual or Pressure Cook timer for 10 minutes. Make sure the timer is set to "Sealing".

3. Once the timer reaches zero, quickly release the pressure. Add heavy cream.

4. Enjoy.

Nutrition: Calories 383, Total Fat 17. 8g, Saturated Fat 10. 1g, Cholesterol 39mg, Sodium 129mg, Total Carbohydrate 44g, Dietary Fiber 2. 4g, Total Sugars 3. 2g, Protein 13. 6g

RECIPES FOR SNACKS

31. Tempeh Patties

Preparation Time: 15 minutes

Cooking Time: 11 minutes

Servings: 5

Ingredients:

- 10 oz tempeh
- 1 carrot, peeled
- 4 tablespoon oatmeal
- 1/4 teaspoon minced garlic
- 1 teaspoon onion powder
- 1/2 teaspoon salt
- 2 oz black beans, canned
- 1 tablespoon tomato sauce
- 1 teaspoon golden syrup
- 1/2 cup water, for cooking

Directions:

1. Cut tempeh into chunks and place it on the steamer rack.

2. Pour water into the instant pot and insert the steamer rack with tempeh.

3. Close the lid and cook on Manual mode (High pressure) for 7 minutes. Then use quick pressure release.

4. Meanwhile, chop the carrot and place it in the food processor.

5. Add minced garlic, oatmeal onion powder, salt, canned beans, tomato sauce, and golden syrup.

6. Blend the mixture for 2-3 minutes.

7. Then add cooked tempeh and keep blending for 1 minute more. The final mixture texture shouldn't be too smooth.

8. Use the burger mold and make burgers. Freeze them until solid.

9. Then wrap every burger in foil or use non-stick paper and place in the cleaned instant pot bowl.

10. Cook the burgers on High (Manual mode) for 4 minutes. Then allow natural pressure release for 10 minutes.

Nutrition: Calories: 175, Fat: 6.6, Fiber: 2.5, Carbs: 18, Protein: 13.7

32. Pumpkin Burgers

Preparation Time: 10 minutes

Cooking Time: 3 minutes

Servings: 2

Ingredients:

- 2 hamburger buns
- 1 tablespoon pumpkin seeds
- 1 tablespoon pumpkin powder
- 3 tablespoon pumpkin puree
- 2 tablespoons breadcrumbs
- 1/2 teaspoon chili flakes
- 1 teaspoon turmeric
- 1 tablespoon flax meal
- 3 tablespoons hot water

Directions:

1. In the mixing bowl combine flax meal and hot water. Whisk the mixture and add pumpkin powder, pumpkin puree, breadcrumbs, chili flakes, and turmeric.
2. Mix up the mixture. Add pumpkin seeds.
3. With the help of the burger mold, make 2 burgers.
4. Place them in the instant pot bowl and close the lid.

5. Set Manual mode (High pressure) and cook for 3 minutes.

6. Then use quick pressure release and open the lid.

7. Fill the burger buns with pumpkin burgers.

Nutrition: Calories: 197, Fat: 5.6, Fiber: 3.3, Carbs: 30.5, Protein: 7.2

33. Fabulous Glazed Carrots

Preparation Time: 15-30 minutes

Cooking Time: 2 hours and 20 minutes

Servings: 5

Ingredients:

- 1 pound of carrots
- 2 teaspoons of chopped cilantro
- 1/4 teaspoon of salt
- 1/4 cup of brown sugar
- 1/4 teaspoon of ground cinnamon
- 1/8 teaspoon of ground nutmeg
- 1 tablespoon of cornstarch
- 1 tablespoon of olive oil
- 2 tablespoons of water
- 1 large orange, juiced and zested

Directions:

1. Peel the carrots, rinse, cut them into 1/4-inch-thick rounds and place them in a 6 quarts slow cooker.
2. Add the salt, sugar, cinnamon, nutmeg, olive oil, orange zest, juice, and stir properly.

3. Cover it with the lid, then plug in the slow cooker and let it cook on the high heat setting for 2 hours or until the carrots become soft.

4. Stir properly the cornstarch and water until it blends well. Thereafter, add this mixture to the slow cooker.

5. Continue cooking for 10 minutes or until the sauce in the slow cooker gets slightly thick.

6. Sprinkle the cilantro over carrots and serve.

Nutrition: Calories:160 Cal, Carbohydrates:40g, Protein:1g, Fats:0. 3g, Fiber:2. 3g.

34. Flavorful Sweet Potatoes with Apples

Preparation Time: 15-30 minutes

Cooking Time: 5 hours

Servings: 6

Ingredients:

- 3 medium-sized apples, peeled and cored
- 6 medium-sized sweet potatoes, peeled and cored
- 1/4 cup of pecans
- 1/4 teaspoon of ground cinnamon
- 1/4 teaspoon of ground nutmeg
- 2 tablespoons of vegan butter, melted
- 1/4 cup of maple syrup

Directions:

1. Cut the sweet potatoes and the apples into 1/2-inch slices.

2. Grease a 6-quarts slow cooker with a non-stick cooking spray and arrange the sweet potato slices in the bottom of the cooker.

3. Top it with the apple slices; sprinkle it with the cinnamon and nutmeg, before garnishing it with butter.

4. Cover it with the lid, plug in the slow cooker and let it cook on the low heat setting for 4 hours or until the sweet potatoes get soft.

5. When done, sprinkle it with pecans and continue cooking for another 30 minutes.

6. Serve right away.

Nutrition: Calories:120 Cal, Carbohydrates:24g, Protein:1g, Fats:3g, Fiber:2g.

35. <u>Buttery Baby Potatoes</u>

Preparation Time: 15-30 minutes

Cooking Time: 40 minutes

Servings: 4

Ingredients:

- 4 tbsp unsalted plant butter, melted
- 4 garlic cloves, minced
- 3 tbsp chopped chives
- Salt and black pepper to taste
- 2 tbsp grated plant-based Parmesan cheese
- 1 ½ lb. baby potatoes, rinsed and drained

Directions:

1. Preheat the oven to 400 F.
2. In a large bowl, mix the butter, garlic, chives, salt, black pepper, and plant Parmesan cheese. Toss the potatoes in the butter mixture until well coated.
3. Spread the mixture into a baking sheet, cover with foil, and roast in the oven for 30 minutes or until tender.
4. Remove the potatoes from the oven and toss in the remaining butter mixture. Serve.

Nutrition: Calories 192 kcal Fats 8.8g Carbs 25.7g Protein 4. 1g

RECIPES FOR SOUP AND STEW

36. Tempeh wild Rice Soup

Preparation Time:05 minutes

Cooking Time: 20 minutes

Servings: 2

Ingredients:

- 1 tablespoon olive oil
- 1 tablespoon coconut flour
- 2 cups vegetable broth or water
- 1cup tempeh
- ¼ cup zucchini diced
- ¼ carrot shredded
- ¼ cup uncooked wild rice
- ¼ tablespoon maple syrup
- 1 teaspoon dried mint
- 1 teaspoon kosher salt
- ½ teaspoon pepper
- 1 clove garlic minced
- 1 teaspoon cilantro chopped for garnish

Directions:

1. Add broth, tempeh, zucchini, carrot, wild rice, maple syrup, mint, salt, pepper, and minced garlic to the Instant Pot and stir to combine. Lock lid, making sure the vent is closed.
2. Using the display panel select the Manual or Pressure Cooker function. Use +/- keys and program the Instant Pot for 15 minutes.
3. When the time is up, let the pressure naturally release for 10 minutes, then quickly release the remaining pressure.
4. In a medium bowl, add coconut flour in olive oil until it makes a paste. Ladle 1 cup of the hot soup broth into the paste and stir to incorporate, then pour flour mixture into the Instant Pot.
5. Using the display panel select Cancel and then Sauté. Cook and stir until thickened, then stir in the half and half.
6. Serve warm topped with chopped cilantro.

Nutrition: Calories 356, Total Fat 17. 8g, Saturated Fat 3.4g, Cholesterol 0mg, Sodium 1957mg, Total Carbohydrate 29 2g, Dietary Fiber 2.7g, Total Sugars 3 9g, Protein 24. 3g

37. Pear Pumpkin Soup

Preparation Time:05 minutes

Cooking Time: 10 minutes

Servings: 2

Ingredients:

- ½ teaspoon butter
- ¼ onion finely diced
- 1 cup pumpkin, peeled and cubed
- 1 pear peeled and cubed
- ½ teaspoon salt
- ¼ teaspoon cumin
- ¼ teaspoon ground coriander
- 1 cup vegetable broth or water
- ½ tablespoon coconut cream
- ½ teaspoon honey

Directions:

1. Add butter to the Instant Pot. Using the display panel select the Sauté function.

2. When butter gets melted, add onions to the Instant Pot and sauté until soft, 2-3 minutes. Add pear, salt, cumin, and spices and stir to combine.

3. Add broth to the Instant Pot then add pumpkin and stir. Turn the Instant Pot off by selecting Cancel, then lock the lid, making sure the vent is closed.

4. Using the display panel select the Manual or Pressure Cooker function. Use the + /- keys and program the Instant Pot for 5 minutes.

5. When the time is up, quickly releasing the remaining pressure, then select Cancel to turn off the pot.

6. Use an immersion blender to blend the soup until smooth.

7. Cool slightly, then stir in coconut cream and honey.

8. Serve warm.

Nutrition: Calories 87, Total Fat 2. 8g, Saturated Fat 1 6g, Cholesterol 3mg, Sodium 972mg, Total Carbohydrate 13. 3g, Dietary Fiber 2 8g, Total Sugars 7.4g, Protein 3. 6g

38. Zucchini Coconut Thai Soup

Preparation Time:15 minutes

Cooking Time: 20 minutes

Servings: 2

Ingredients:

- ½ tablespoon olive oil
- ½ onion, peeled and diced
- ½ pound zucchini, peeled and diced
- 1 cup spinach
- 1 small carrot
- 1 teaspoon ginger garlic paste
- ½ tablespoon red curry paste
- 2 cups vegetable broth or water
- ½ teaspoon maple syrup
- ½ cup coconut milk canned
- 1 tablespoon lime juice
- 1/4 teaspoon red pepper flakes
- 1 teaspoon of sea salt
- 1/2 teaspoon black pepper ground
- 1/4 cup basil

Directions:

1. Press the Sauté button on the Instant Pot. When the display shows "Hot", add olive oil and heat it.

2. Add the onions and carrots, zucchinis, spinach. Sauté for 3–5 minutes until onions are translucent.

3. Add the ginger-garlic paste and curry paste. Continue to sauté for 1 minute.

4. Add remaining ingredients, except basil. Lock lid.

5. Press the Soup button and set the time to 20 minutes. When the timer beeps, let the pressure release naturally for 10 minutes. Quickly release any additional pressure until the float valve drops and then unlock the lid.

6. In the Instant Pot, puree soup with a hand blender, or use a stand blender and puree in batches.

7. Ladle into bowls, garnish each bowl with basil, and serve hot.

8. Have fun!

Nutrition: Calories 136, Total Fat 7 2g, Saturated Fat 2.1g, Cholesterol 0mg, Sodium 1930mg, Total Carbohydrate 11.8g, Dietary Fiber 2 3g, Total Sugars 5.7g, Protein 7g

39. <u>Vegetable and Cottage Cheese Soup</u>

Preparation Time:35 minutes

Cooking Time: 15 minutes

Servings: 2

Ingredients:

- ½ package cottage cheese, drained and cut into ¾-inch cubes
- 1 tablespoon coconut oil
- ½ teaspoon dried Italian seasoning
- 1 diced tomato
- 1 cup vegetable broth
- ½ cup fresh peas
- ½ cup kale
- ¼ cup cauliflower
- ½ cup 1-inch pieces green beans
- ½ cup chopped green sweet pepper
- ¼ cup sliced green olives

Directions:

1. Put the cottage cheese in a plastic bag within a flat plate. Add the oil and Italian seasoning; Turn to cover the cottage cheese. Marinate in the refrigerator for 2 to 4 hours.

2. Press the Sauté button on the Instant Pot. When the display shows "Hot", add coconut oil and heat it. Press Sauté function and add cottage cheese and set timer for 5 minutes until cottage cheese browns.

3. Add broth and tomato into IP. Then Add peas, kale, cauliflower, green beans, green sweet pepper, and green olives and again set the timer for 10 minutes and lock the lid of Instant Pot.

4. When time is up, let the pressure release naturally for 10 minutes. Quickly release any additional pressure until the float valve drops and then unlock the lid.

5. Serve the soup and enjoy.

Nutrition: Calories229, Total Fat 12.3g, Saturated Fat 8.6g, Cholesterol 13mg, Sodium 765mg, Total Carbohydrate 16.9g, Dietary Fiber 4.5g, Total Sugars 6. 4g, Protein 15g

40. <u>Zucchini Tomato Soup</u>

Preparation Time:15 minutes

Cooking Time: 15 minutes

Servings: 2

Ingredients:

- 1-pound large tomatoes, cored and cut into pieces
- ¼ zucchini, cut into chunks
- ¼ cup broccoli
- 1 medium bell pepper, seeded and cut into pieces
- 1 teaspoon garlic powder
- 2 tablespoons butter, divided
- 1 tablespoon vinegar, divided
- 1 teaspoon plus a pinch of salt, divided
- ½ teaspoon plus a pinch of ground pepper, divided
- ¼ avocado
- ¼ tablespoon chopped fresh basil
- Enough water

Directions:

1. Cut all the vegetables and set them aside.
2. Press the Sauté mode and pour in the butter. When it melts, add zucchini, broccoli, and bell pepper and mix

them. Sauté for a few minutes or until the vegetables are tender, about 5 minutes.

3. Add garlic powder, water, and spices and mix.

4. lock lid. Set Manual cook or Pressure for 4 minutes on High Pressure.

5. Allow the IP to Natural-release for 5 minutes once the timer goes off.

6. Remove the lid and mix well. Serve soup with a topping of avocado and fresh basil.

7. Have fun!

Nutrition: Calories 228, Total Fat 17. 1g, Saturated Fat 8 4g, Cholesterol 31mg, Sodium 1266mg, Total Carbohydrate 18.5g, Dietary Fiber 6.1g, Total Sugars 10.1g, Protein 4. 1g

RECIPES FOR SALAD

41. Parsley Chard Salad

Preparation time: 10 minutes

Cooking time: 0 minutes

Servings: 4

Ingredients:

- 1-pound red chard, steamed and torn
- 1 cup grapes, halved
- 1 cup cherry tomatoes, halved
- 1 celery stalk, chopped
- 3 tablespoons balsamic vinegar
- ½ cup coconut cream
- 1 teaspoon chili powder
- 2 tablespoons olive oil
- ½ cup parsley, minced
- A pinch of sea salt and black pepper

Directions:

1. In a bowl, combine the chard with the grapes, tomatoes and the other Ingredient, toss and serve right away.

Nutrition: calories 250, fat 4, fiber 8, carbs 20, protein 6.5

42. Tomato Cucumber Cheese Salad

Preparation time: 15 minutes

Cooking time: 15 minutes

Servings: 2

Ingredients:

- 2 cups tomatoes, sliced
- 2 cucumbers, peeled, sliced
- 2 spring onions, sliced
- 7-ounces mozzarella cheese, chopped
- 12 black olives
- 2 teaspoons basil pesto
- 2 tablespoons extra-virgin olive oil
- 2 tablespoons basil, fresh, chopped

Directions:

1. In a large salad bowl, add basil pesto and cheese. Mix well. Add remaining Ingredients into a bowl and toss to blend. Serve fresh and enjoy!

Nutritional Values (Per Serving): Calories: 609 Fat: 50.5 g Carbohydrates: 13.7 g Sugar: 7.5 g Protein: 27.2 g Cholesterol: 47 mg

43. Healthy Brussels Sprout Salad

Preparation time: 15 minutes

Cooking time: 10 minutes

Servings: 1

Ingredients:

- ½ teaspoon apple cider vinegar
- 6 Brussels sprouts, washed, sliced
- 1 tablespoon Parmesan cheese, fresh, grated
- 1 teaspoon extra-virgin olive oil
- ¼ teaspoon pepper
- ¼ teaspoon sea salt

Directions:

1. Add all your Ingredients into a large salad bowl, toss to blend. Serve and enjoy!

Nutritional Values (Per Serving): Calories: 156 Fat: 9.6 g Carbohydrates: 10.7 g Sugar: 2.5 g Cholesterol: 10 mg Protein: 10

44. Chickpea Salad

Preparation time: 20 minutes

Cooking time: 25 minutes

Servings: 5

Ingredients:

- 1 cup chickpea
- 1 red onion, sliced
- ½ cup fresh parsley, chopped
- 1 tablespoon olive oil
- 1 teaspoon salt
- 3 cups vegetable broth
- 1 teaspoon garam masala

Directions:

1. Place chickpeas and vegetable broth in the instant pot. Add garam masala.
2. Close and seal the lid. Set High-pressure mode and cook chickpeas for 25 minutes.
3. After this, allow naturally pressure release for 10 minutes.
4. In the salad bowl combine together cooked chickpeas, chopped parsley, sliced onion, salt, and olive oil.
5. Mix up the salad carefully before serving.

Nutrition: calories 184, fat 5.3, fiber 7.8, carbs 27.3, protein 8.2

45. <u>Lentil Tomato Salad</u>

Preparation time: 10 minutes

Cooking time: 7 minutes

Servings: 5

Ingredients:

- 2 cups baby spinach
- 1 cup lentils
- 2 cups of water
- 1 teaspoon salt
- 1 teaspoon ground black pepper
- 3 tomatoes, chopped
- 1 red onion, sliced
- 2 tablespoons olive oil
- 1 tablespoon lemon juice

Directions:

1. Cook lentils: mix up lentils, water, and salt. Transfer the mixture in the instant pot.

2. Close and seal the lid and cook on Manual for 7 minutes. Then use quick pressure release.

3. Meanwhile, make all the remaining Preparations combine together baby spinach with tomatoes, and red onion in the salad bowl.

4. Sprinkle with lemon juice, olive oil, and ground black pepper. Don't stir the salad.

5. Chill the cooked lentils till the room temperature and add in the salad bowl.

6. Mix up the cooked meal carefully and serve it warm.

Nutrition: calories 210, fat 6.3, fiber 13.5, carbs 28.8, protein 11.2

RECIPES FOR DESSERT

46. Egg Custard

Preparation Time: 10 minutes

Cooking Time: 40 minutes

Serve: 6

Ingredients:

- 3 eggs
- 2 egg yolks
- 1/2 tsp vanilla
- 1 tsp ground nutmeg
- 1/2 cup erythritol
- 2 cups heavy whipping cream

Directions:

1. Preheat the oven to 350 F.
2. In a mixing bowl, whisk together all ingredients until just combined.
3. Pour mixture into the glass pie dish and bake for 40 minutes.
4. Allow to cool completely then place in the refrigerator for 2 hours.
5. Serve chilled and enjoy.

Nutrition: Calories 190 Fat 18.6 g Carbohydrates 1.7 g Sugar 0.4 g Protein 4.5 g Cholesterol 207 mg

47. <u>Frozen Vanilla Custard</u>

Preparation Time: 10 minutes

Cooking Time: 15 minutes

Serve: 4

Ingredients:

- 4 eggs, separated
- 1/4 tsp cream of tartar
- 1/2 tsp vanilla
- 1 tsp liquid stevia
- 4 oz butter, unsalted
- 4 oz mascarpone cheese

Direction:

1. In a saucepan, heat butter, cheese, and egg yolk over low heat until thickened. Whisk constantly.
2. Remove from heat. Stir in vanilla and sweetener.
3. In a separate bowl, beat egg whites and cream of tartar until stiff.
4. Fold egg white mixture into the egg yolk mixture. Pour mixture into the container and place it in the freezer for 1 hour.

5. Pour custard mixture into the ice cream machine and churn according to machine instructions until get desired consistency.

6. Serve and enjoy.

Nutrition: Calories 318 Fat 31 g Carbohydrates 1.4 g Sugar 0.5 g Protein 9 g Cholesterol 239 mg

48. Easy Chocolate Frosty

Preparation Time: 10 minutes

Cooking Time: 10 minutes

Serve: 4

Ingredients:

- 1 cup heavy whipping cream
- 5 drops liquid stevia
- 1 tsp vanilla
- 1 tbsp almond butter
- 2 tbsp unsweetened cocoa powder

Directions:

1. Add heavy whipping cream into the medium bowl and beat using the hand mixer for 5 minutes.
2. Add remaining ingredients and blend until thick whipped cream form.
3. Pour in serving bowls and place them in the freezer for 30 minutes.
4. Serve and enjoy.

Nutrition: Calories 137 Fat 13.7 g Carbohydrates 3.2 g Sugar 0.4 g Protein 2 g Cholesterol 41 mg

49. Easy Berry Ice Cream

Preparation Time: 10 minutes

Cooking Time: 10 minutes

Serve: 6

Ingredients:

- 2/3 cup heavy cream
- 2 tbsp Swerve
- 10 oz frozen berries

Directions:

1. Add frozen berries and Swerve into the food processor and process until just berries are chopped.
2. Add heavy cream and process until smooth.
3. Serve immediately and enjoy it.

Nutrition: Calories 75 Fat 5.1 g Carbohydrates 6.8 g Sugar 3.4 g Protein 0.6 g Cholesterol 18 mg

50. <u>Frozen Whips</u>

Preparation Time: 10 minutes

Cooking Time: 10 minutes

Serve: 12

Ingredients:

- 1 cup heavy whipping cream
- 1/2 tsp vanilla
- 2 1/2 tbsp Swerve
- 4 tbsp unsweetened cocoa powder
- Pinch of salt

Directions:

1. Line baking sheet with parchment paper and set aside.
2. Add heavy whipping cream into the large mixing bowl. Add remaining ingredients and stir well.
3. Using a hand mixer beat heavy cream mixture until firm peaks form.
4. Transfer cream mixture into the piping bag. On the prepared baking sheet swirl the cream around into large mounds. Make 12 cream mounds.
5. Place the baking sheet in the freezer for 1 hour.
6. Serve and enjoy.

Nutrition: Calories 40 Fat 4 g Carbohydrates 1.7 g Sugar 0.1 g
Protein 0.6 g Cholesterol 14 mg

CONCLUSION

tart with the remark below if you wish to plan a picnic for two people. You may find this to be helpful if you are struggling with which ingredients to buy for your next meal. It also includes a list of cookbooks that you can purchase from a bookstore or online. I hope you'll be able to discover something you enjoy!

Note: One serving = 6 or 8 ounces of cooked meat, fish, or poultry; 2 ounces of nuts, seeds, dairy, and eggs; 1 cup vegetables or salad; and 1/2 of a cup of cooked grains.

1. Your salad should include lots of greens such as spinach (spinach is the most nutritious), kale (kale is more nutritious than spinach. You can use other types of greens too depending on what you get at the supermarket.), chard (very nutritious), arugula (very nutritious), and lettuce. I recommend eating at least two big salads each day. Hummus is popular, but I suggest it is better for you to use avocado or a nut/seed spread (if you eat nuts & seeds) instead. I would also suggest eating some pumpkin seeds (they are a great source of protein) and sunflower seeds (a good source of fat). You can also use Nuts & Seed Oils or Nut Butter on your salad or sandwich.

2. If you buy some meat, salmon is an excellent choice because high in heart-healthy omega-3 fatty acids and low in calories. For some reason, most people do not eat enough fish, so I would recommend eating at least one serving per day. Other choices include chicken and turkey. If you do eat beef, try to buy the lean cuts of beef. In some cases, you can buy ground skinless chicken or turkey breast. If you cannot find it in your store, you can use a third-party source.

3. I would not recommend eating nuts and seeds on a daily basis if you do not eat them on a regular basis. At most, eat them two or three times each week. Buy raw ones if possible because they are more nutritious and their natural oils (especially flax seeds oil) are still intact. Make sure that your nuts or seeds are fresh by checking the expiration date before buying them from the supermarket or a third-party source (eBay, Amazon). If you do not like store-bought nuts, you can make your own nut butter (ground almonds or walnuts are good too).

4. If you are making a salad, buy some dried cranberries, strawberries (fresh or dried), and/or apples. If you want to use regular apples, I suggest you buy Gala or Fuji apples because they are sweet. Other types of apples such as Braeburns and

Red Delicious are not that sweet. Be careful: some people may be allergic to apple seeds which contain a chemical called amygdalin (this chemical can turn into cyanide in the body). Therefore, do not eat the seeds if it is possible because it would be better for your health.

5. Cheese is good to eat if you do not have a dairy allergy. Some types of cheese are high in sodium, so be careful if you do not like salty food.

6. If you have some nuts, seeds, and/or avocados left after making your sandwiches, I suggest you make this recipe: (Cut the recipe in half or even quarter it for 1 serving).

Lightning Source UK Ltd.
Milton Keynes UK
UKHW022158190821
389154UK00002B/315